Advance praise

"I've had the pleasure of meeting Morgan and her family. She is an inspiring young woman whose insight into her Type 1 diabetes will help others, and their families, to confront the vulnerabilities of the disease. Readers will learn from Morgan how to manage these issues with composure and strength."

—**Robin Roberts**, Co-Anchor Good Morning America

"I have had the opportunity to review many manuscripts about diabetes and this is one of the very best. Ms. Panzirer is a talented writer and is able to describe the technical aspects of living with diabetes quite adeptly. But the heart of this book is her journey, how she describes meeting with President Obama, Pope Francis and competing in high level equestrian competition within the context of the grinding self discipline required to maintain her diabetes. There is no self-pity, just a full-on attitude of living a fantastic life in spite of, or because of, having Type 1 diabetes and inspiring others to do the same."

—**Dr. Anne Peters,** Director, USC Westside Center for Diabetes, Professor, Keck School of Medicine of USC, Director, USC Clinical Diabetes Programs

"Optimism and determination in the face of a challenge is a potent combination. Morgan Panzirer, when faced with Type 1 diabetes at the age of six, saw the glass half full and challenges that she would overcome. Can she? Heck yeah she can and she has! Morgan is a Type 1 Diabetes Champion and an inspiration."

—**Aaron Kowalski**, CEO of JDRF

"Morgan is an inspiring young lady whose insight into her Type 1 diabetes will help others, and their families, to confront the vulnerabilities of the disease and learn to manage them with composure and strength. She teaches us through her writing how to deal with the emotional, as well as medical, aspects of the disease using humor and blunt honesty."

—**Robin Smith**, President of The Stem For Life Foundation

"OK, here's the deal, having Type 1 diabetes s*#@s. She'd never admit it, but I'm pretty sure that's how Morgan would describe it…at least at the beginning. What I took away from *Actually, I Can* was not the charmed life, meeting celebrities and traveling the world. It was that after confronting the awfulness of her diagnosis, Morgan was able to face her disease and take control of it, including the difficult, painful ups and downs. In my decades as a journalist I've learned that there's absolutely no substitute for hearing about a disease from someone who's walked in those shoes. In *Actually, I Can* Morgan describes to both young T1D children and their parents that while diabetes is undoubtedly a challenge, it can be managed and be something that doesn't s*#@ nearly so much."

—**Dr. Max Gomez**, Emmy-award winning medical correspondent and senior health editor for NBC

"Morgan is a fellow T1D teammate of mine and her book is about life with this challenging disease. But instead of bringing her down, the condition brings out the best in her amazing inner character and great sense of humor (or wit). With unstoppable perseverance to overcome all obstacles, Morgan turns this setback into an advantage and lives her life with no regrets. It is awesome to hear her perspective and to see another person with T1D thrive while managing all the disease throws at her on a daily basis. Very Inspirational! *This is a must read!* In the end, the only thing T1D does to us is make us stronger."

—**Max Domi**, Author of *No Days Off: My Life with Type 1 Diabetes and Journey to the NHL*

"Morgan has an authentic voice in the diabetes patient perspective. She unabashedly stares down and addresses the unrelenting challenges one faces in diabetes diagnosis and management, sans sugarcoating. Accompanied by gritty optimism, her impressive insight on progressing diabetes research, emerging tech and medications will impress readers with a resilient hope that a fulfilled and healthy life is possible."

—**Gary Hall, Jr.**, first Olympian/Gold Medalist with Type One Diabetes, Olympic Hall of Fame, 10 x Medals in Swimming, Patient Advocate

"Many books have been written about children and teenagers with Type 1 diabetes. What makes *Actually, I Can* unique—and groundbreaking—is that the author is herself a teenager. Morgan Panzirer was diagnosed at age six and, in a voice that is authentic and unflinching, she describes the realities of growing up with Type 1:

the stresses and the setbacks, and also the small triumphs and the life-long lessons. This is a story about family, faith, and friendships, and includes remarkable encounters with politicians, pop stars, and even the Pope. Every teenager with diabetes should read this book. So, too, should their parents and their health care providers as well. A triumph."

—**Kelly L. Close**, founder, diaTribe.org

"Morgan Panzirer wants to be a pediatric endocrinologist. Sign me up! I'm no longer a kid, but after reading her book, I know that Morgan will bring wisdom, empathy, and love—and a trove of experience—to whatever she does in her life. *Actually, I Can* taught me a lot about Morgan. Growing up with Type 1 diabetes, she's already faced skeptics who doubt she will realize all of her dreams. Actually, she can, and she will."

—**James S. Hirsch**, author, best-selling *Cheating Destiny*

Actually,
I Can.

Actually, I Can.

GROWING UP WITH **TYPE 1 DIABETES**,
A STORY OF UNEXPECTED EMPOWERMENT

Morgan J. Panzirer

T1D Media
NEW YORK

Actually, I Can.

Growing Up with Type 1 Diabetes, A Story of Unexpected Empowerment

Morgan J. Panzirer

ISBN: 978-0-578-65393-8

Library of Congress Control Number: 2020908785

Medical Disclaimers: Although the author and publisher have made every effort to ensure that the information in this book was correct at press time, the author and publisher do not assume and hereby disclaim any liability to any party for any loss, damage, or disruption caused by errors or omissions, whether such errors or omissions result from negligence, accident, or any other cause. This book is not intended to provide any medical advice. The reader should consult a physician in matters relating to health and particularly with respect to any symptoms that may require diagnosis or medical attention.

Published by T1D Media

T1D Media
NEW YORK

Dedication

I dedicate this book to my family.
Mom, Dad, Caroline, and Luke: thank you for
helping me through this rollercoaster ride
and being there every step of the way.
I cannot thank you enough for never giving up
and always being so supportive of me.
I love you all more than you will ever know.

And to all of my fellow Type 1 diabetics,
keep fighting and dream on!

Table of Contents

PART IV

PART V

PART VI

Prologue

Before I start, I figured it would be a good idea for you to get to know me a little bit. So first off, hello! (Cue the Adele song here. Sorry, I'm kind of a huge fan of hers.) My name is Morgan and I'm from Katonah, New York which is a small town about forty miles north of New York City. I have an awesome family. It consists of my mom, Karen, my dad, David, my sister, Caroline, and my brother, Luke. I am the oldest. Caroline is three years younger than I am followed by Luke, who is six years younger than me. And of course, my three dogs, Parker, Owen, and Marshall.

I am also a huge fan of school. Right about now you're probably thinking, "This girl is crazy, (and such a nerd!). She actually enjoys school?" That would be three yeses: I am crazy, I do love school, and I am a nerd. The whole learning aspect of it is pretty neat. Okay, I'll stop now before you think I'm even nerdier than you already do. Anyway, I go to Villanova University and I am a biology major with a minor in Spanish literature and language, and I'm hoping to go to medical school after college.

Hmmm, what else? Well I feel like I should say something about what motivated me to write this book. One day, I picked up Ellen DeGeneres' book called, *Seriously, I'm Kidding.* I started reading it and loved the way she wrote. I had begun writing this book a year prior, and decided, what the heck? Maybe I should finish it. I wrote for about a year and a half and then pushed it aside and didn't look at it for almost four years. One day I was just opening random files on my computer and found it. I decided that I wanted to edit and finish it because there are so many people out there who need to be educated about Type 1 diabetes and its seriousness.

I'm also an avid horseback rider. I have a horse named Gideon (no I did not name him) and I ride on the Villanova University Equestrian Team. Oh, and one of my biggest pet peeves is…no, I don't race (which is what everyone asks!). I do the hunter divisions. For you non-horse people, I'll keep it short and sweet…Gideon and I jump over jumps.

That's pretty much my life in a nutshell. School and riding. Seems boring right now, but trust me, when I tell you about the component that was added in 2007, I will have a lot more stories to tell. Oh, and there's one more thing you should know about me before I start telling you about my journey thus far…I am extremely sarcastic. So the bottom line is, don't get confused if I am being my usual sarcastic self.

Part I

"Life is not about waiting for the storm to pass. It's about learning how to dance in the rain."

ANONYMOUS

The Diagnosis

I was diagnosed with Type 1 diabetes one month after my sixth birthday. At the time, I had a three-year-old sister and a three-month-old brother, so as you can imagine my parents already had their hands full. Prior to my diagnosis, my dad worked in the commercial real estate industry in New York City and my mom was a nutritionist.

It all began when one day, my mom noticed I was drinking and peeing a lot. She knew this was one of the signs of being a Type 1 diabetic from her prior experience as a nutritionist. She brought a urine sample to my pediatrician and said, "I'm sure it's nothing. But humor me and test it anyway." Sure enough, a few days later a phone call came to my mom while we were driving in the car. One that, little she did know, would change all of our lives forever.

When my mom picked up the phone to answer the call she was fine, thinking nothing of it at all. She thought the doctor was going to call to tell her that everything came back negative and sure enough, she was in fact overreacting. However, when she picked up the phone, my pediatrician came on the other line and said to my mom, "Karen, I have no idea how to tell you this…but Morgan has Type 1 diabetes. I made an appointment for you tomorrow at the Naomi Berrie Diabetes Center at Columbia. Plan to spend the day. I'm so sorry."

When I was thirteen I wrote, *I remember being in the car with my mom when she hung up the phone and immediately started crying. That was the moment that reality had set in; her oldest daughter was a Type 1 diabetic. And unfortunately she knew exactly what that meant. A life of not being a normal six-year-old anymore. A life of becoming a pancreas. A life of pricking her daughter's fingers fifteen times a day and injecting insulin several more to attempt to keep her blood sugars stable. All of this, just to keep her child alive. You can imagine the amount of pressure my parents felt. Needless to say, it was a tough couple of weeks to follow to say the least.*

Now looking back at this life-altering event, I am finally able to see the incredibly important life lesson that my diagnosis taught me. I had always been a generally happy person who just wanted to enjoy life, but I experienced firsthand how the course of one's life can change in an instant. That one phone call changed not only my life, but my family members' lives as well. Literally two minutes prior my mom and I were smiling and just enjoying the day, but that one forty-second conversation changed absolutely everything. We have one chance to thrive on this Earth that, right now, we call home. But one day we won't have that privilege anymore. The scary but important part to note about this is that we have no idea if that day is today or thirty years from now, so we need to appreciate every single second. Each one is truly a gift.

The Basics

As I just mentioned, in 2007 when I was six years old I faced a devastating Type 1 diabetes diagnosis. Type 1 is an autoimmune disease where a person's pancreas stops producing insulin, a hormone that enables us to get energy from food. (If you don't know what I mean by "autoimmune disease," then Google it. No don't, I'm kidding. Just keep reading. It basically means my own body attacked and killed the insulin-producing beta cells in my pancreas).

In school, I often hear health teachers trying to explain to students what "diabetes" is. Don't get me wrong, I think it's great that they are trying to inform kids about it but there's one problem: there are two types and it is not acceptable to lump them together.

More frequently than you would think people say, "Oh diabetes is when you are overweight, don't exercise, and don't eat healthy foods. You just take your insulin and you're fine." That is three big fat no's and quite simply incorrect. Especially for Type 1. Not even close.

The majority of the time, Type 1 and Type 2 diabetes get

lumped into just "diabetes" which is problematic. Type 2 can be cured and/or managed by taking a pill (or in some cases one shot a day), exercising, and eating better. However, there is no cure for Type 1 diabetes. With Type 1, I essentially need to act as a pancreas at all times. I am constantly being monitored. No breaks. No vacations. This disease is 24/7, 365 days per year. It is a chronic illness that affects everything I do, and every decision I make. Anything from a little cold to being angry about doing poorly on a test affects my blood sugar. It is a constant battle that never ends. The part that's so frustrating about it, is that the only thing consistent with Type 1 is the inconsistency (kudos to my dad for that line). Nothing is ever the same day to day. It is also an extremely dangerous disease. As my dad always says, "It's the only disease I know of where the same drug that is keeping you alive can also kill you by the slightest overdose."

Just so you get a sense of the numbers, a "good" blood glucose level is anywhere from 80-130mg/dL. Under 80mg/dL is getting into the low range and over 130mg/dL gets into the high range. You feel like crap when your blood sugar is either high or low. Different people feel differently, but for me there really isn't one that I can say is worse than the other. They both completely and utterly suck.

If you yourself don't have Type 1, you're probably wondering how it feels to have a high or low blood sugar. When I'm low, I start shaking and sweating uncontrollably. I get super fatigued and exhausted, almost like I have the flu. But the scary part is that I never know whether I feel tired because I'm low and am about to faint, or if I am just flat-out tired.

If I had to sum up being low in a few terms, it honestly feels like you are about to die (I understand that that sounds really harsh, but I can assure you that I'm not exaggerating). As for high, I don't usually get any symptoms unless I've been in the high range for an extended period of time whereas you get symptoms from being low instantly. (By extended period of time I mean a couple of hours). At that point I get really angry, cranky, and tired. I usually get migraines, too, which sucks, as I'm sure you know if you've ever experienced one. When I'm extremely high for an extended period of time (we're talking over 300mg/dL), I feel exhausted and I start throwing up. It's not a fun experience, trust me. Being low and high are both really dangerous if not handled in a timely manner. When low, one is prone to seizures and if low enough, death. When high for a long period of time, one is prone to DKA or, diabetic ketoacidosis. DKA is extremely serious and often causes patients to be in a coma or even die.

When I was diagnosed, my blood sugar was 600mg/dL. My mom thinks I went into a comatose state at night because every night for three weeks before I was diagnosed, I would sleepwalk downstairs into my parents' bedroom and just stare at my mom. I wouldn't say anything. She thinks it was my way of telling her something was wrong because I couldn't verbalize it. She said when it happened she would bring me to the bathroom, I would pee and then she'd put me back to sleep in my bed. I give my mom a lot of credit because if my child walked into my room sleep-walking with his/her eyes blankly staring at me, I would be very creeped out. Just thinking about it gives me the chills. It's just so weird.

Type 1 diabetes is thought to possibly have a genetic component and is completely unpreventable. In my case, we do not think it was genetic, but are not entirely sure given one of the events that happened later on in my life. There is no trace of Type 1 diabetes in my family. I am just one of the lucky people who gets to deal with this awesome disease (notice the sarcasm is starting)...every single day.

P.S. - I can eat sugar!!!

P.P.S. - I can eat anything I want and it doesn't have to be sugar-free as long as I give myself the proper amount of insulin. There is no special diet I have to follow. I can eat literally anything I want to. Sorry, that sounds super aggressive but I can't tell you how many times people assume everything I eat has to be sugar-free. It is incredibly frustrating.

P.P.P.S. - I don't have to eat on a special schedule. I can eat whenever I want just like you.

In short, if there is one thing you take away from this book, I hope it's that people with Type 1 can eat sugar and do not have to follow a diet. I'm joking...there's a bunch of things I want you to take away from this book, but the fact that I can eat sugar is one of the important ones.

Gadgets

I'm sure the suspense is killing you (or you may be like, why am I still reading?) but I need to address one last thing before we officially get started for the third time (in case you couldn't tell I get side-tracked. A lot). Many people get confused when they see "gadgets" (or as some say, the spy gear and/or 3D stickers…don't ask - I've heard it all!) attached to my body so I figured I would explain that and the terminology before we officially get started. Besides, I use terms like "CGM" and "pod" a lot so you should probably know what they mean.

I wear two gadgets on my body. I will start with my insulin pump or as I refer to it, the pod. It is actually called the OmniPod but it's just easier to say "pod." This is a small, rectangular sort of white box with adhesive underneath (it looks kind of like a computer mouse) that is attached to me, and, before you ask, yes there is a needle that stays in me at all times. Well, technically speaking it's a tiny blue plastic canula through which the needle initially shoots in and comes out, leaving the canula behind, but you know what I mean.

The canula is like a very thin straw. In layman's terms, I inject insulin into a little hole on the pod which then delivers it by the hour based on how I program the pump. This little bit every hour is known as basal (no, not the plant which is spelled basil. However, they are pronounced the same). Then, when I eat or my blood sugar is high, I manually program in how many grams of carbohydrates I am eating or what my blood sugar is, and then the pod delivers insulin to me via the canula.

Because I just told you that I get side-tracked a lot, I'm going to take it upon myself to tell you a funny story about "grams" of carbs. The day after I was diagnosed, I went into New York City to a Type 1 diabetes center where we spent the day learning about my new life (I'll get into the details later). While my parents and I were sitting in the endocrinologist's office, he was telling us all about grams of carbs and how many I should eat when my blood sugar is a certain number. Well me being a little six-year-old with an enormous appetite, I was certain that he was telling me I got to eat fifteen graham crackers when my blood sugar was 65 mg/dL and twenty when it was 50 mg/dL. I thought it seemed like a lot but hey, I got to eat graham crackers all of the time! How bad could that be? I learned later it could be pretty bad; especially when those grams you're eating aren't graham crackers.

Okay sorry, back to the technical stuff…I have become really good at estimating how many carbs are in any given food because most of the things I eat do not have food labels. For example, I can look at a cupcake and estimate how many carbs are in it according to the amount of frosting, size of it, etc. Although people generally think of sugar being the thing people with "diabetes" need to concern themselves with, this is actually a little misleading. For example, Dr. Anne Peters conducted a study that showed whether you eat a piece of chocolate cake or a baked potato, the post prandial glucose response is the same.

I switch the pod's location every three days for two reasons: 1) I need to refill the insulin chamber so I don't run out and die and 2) I have to move it to different parts of my body so scar tissue doesn't build up.

It was difficult learning to use the pod. I'll never forget the time I went into New York City to get my pump (not the same day I mixed up grams and grahams). I spent an entire day trying to understand which button meant what and when to use them all. The buttons on it have the ability to kill me, and that was nerve-racking to wrap my head around at six years old. Talk about a lot of pressure!

Now for my CGM or, continuous glucose monitor. This is an oval shaped plastic piece containing a gray transmitter. It has a wire about an inch and a half long coming out of the end, which is what stays inside of me. The purpose of this one is to test my blood sugar every five minutes and give me a trend of where it's heading. The awesome part about the CGM is that it eliminates the need to prick my finger as frequently as I would have to do normally. Without it, I test my blood sugar (by pricking my finger) about ten to fifteen times per day, versus only two or three with using it. So you can see what a huge impact it has on my everyday life. My blood sugar readings go directly to my phone which is pretty amazing. The not-so-cool part is that it also goes to my parents' phones which only means that they text me nonstop to see if I have corrected a high or low blood sugar. It gets really annoying but I know they are just trying to look out for me. You would think they trust me by now considering I've been dealing with this for over ten years. Anyway, I change the CGM's location on my body every ten days to avoid scar tissue buildup, but also because the sensor expires after that time.

Thinking back now to the days where CGMs were still being engineered and developed, I honestly don't know how I lived without one. I remember every time I went to the endocrinologist he would ask to look at my fingertips because he was afraid I was losing feeling in my fingers from pricking them so often. For a solid eight years of my life, I lived with hundreds of little black dots on my finger tips from all of the needles. But it wasn't like I had a choice. It's pretty incredible that in a relatively short period of time the technology has gotten significantly better; and I'm sure soon enough I'll be saying, "I don't know how I ever lived without *insert name of new life-changing technology here.*"

Also a quick side note because people generally get confused as to how I shower…these two devices are waterproof so I don't have to take them off to swim, shower, or do whatever other water activities one may do in his/her daily life. However, the pumps that are connected via tubing are not waterproof, so there is a little clip that you can undo which leaves the canula in your body, but just detaches the pump itself. This essentially means that you are getting no insulin while your pump is disconnected.

Bottom line is, if you see people walking around on the street with what looks like spy gear attached to them, please don't stare. Chances are it's probably someone like me who is just wearing these weird-looking things to stay alive!

Technicalities

There are so many little things that go into living with Type 1. Both people who use and don't use a pump have to put a lot of thought into every decision they make. Whether it is the math required to count carbs or trying to understand a trend, it is a ton of thought. One aspect of life with Type 1 that probably took me the longest to figure out is programming my pump and all of the various settings.

Just in case you haven't gone through the stress and frustration of programming an insulin pump, I figured I would walk you through the different settings and what they all mean. There are three different parts to the job. The first is what we call "insulin-to-carb ratios." What these ratios represent is basically how many carbs I can eat per unit of insulin. I'll give you an example just so you get a better idea. I'm eating a cupcake and based on my high-tech carb estimation program (also known as my brain), I think it looks to be about thirty grams of carbs. If my insulin-to-carb ratio is set at ten grams, I would need three units of insulin in order to keep my blood sugar stable. This seems pretty easy just thinking about it, but it takes a lot of trial and error to figure out what the correct ratios actually are. They also vary based on the time of day. For me, my insulin-to-carb (IC) ratio is lower for breakfast than it is for dinner. It will sound a little bit backwards, but a lower IC ratio means that I can eat fewer grams of carbs per unit of insulin. So if I were to eat that same thirty-gram cupcake for breakfast, I would get more insulin than if I ate it for dessert.

The next part of pump programming that we need to concern ourselves with is correction factors. These are fairly similar to IC ratios. They are the number of points in mg/dL that my blood sugar will drop per unit (U) of insulin. These depend on what my "target blood glucose" is set at. Generally, I have it set to 100mg/dL. This may seem confusing, so let me give you a hypothetical situation. My blood sugar is 200mg/dL and my correction factor is 25mg/dL/U. If I want to go down one hundred points because my target is set at 100mg/dL, I would need four units of insulin (25mg/dL * 4 units of insulin = drop by 100mg/dL). Again, these correction factors are also sensitive to the time of day. For me specifically, my correction factors are lower during the night than they are during the day. Like IC ratios, it sounds a little bit backwards, but a lower correction factor means more insulin. So to drop my blood glucose by one hundred points at 12am would take more insulin than it would to drop the same one hundred points at 2pm. This discrepancy is mainly due to hormones. Hormone levels are generally greater overnight, which makes my blood sugars trend higher. This explains why both my IC ratios and correction factors are lower at night.

The final part of programming is basal rates. As I mentioned briefly back in the beginning, basal is a specific amount of insulin that is delivered automatically by the pump every hour (it's measured in units of insulin per hour). People who don't wear a pump get this little bit every hour through an injection known as long-acting insulin. They do this injection once daily and it slowly gets absorbed into the bloodstream, making a little bit of it get released throughout the day. This functions the same way basal rates on the pump do. Basal rates are extremely time sensitive. To give you an idea, I have eleven different basal settings in my pump. I have a different basal rate for the following times: 12am, 2am, 3am, 5am, 9am, 12pm, 3pm, 5pm, 6pm, 8pm, and 10pm. My basal is the highest at night, again because of all of the different hormones.

The difficult part about programming a pump, is it's not like you do it once and then you're good. I have to constantly be looking at the trends on my continuous glucose monitor to figure out where and what I can adjust. For example, if I was low for three days in a row after eating lunch, I was most likely getting too much insulin for lunch, meaning I need to increase my IC ratio for lunchtime. On the other hand, if I hadn't eaten anything and I woke up low at 7am for a couple of days, I can assume that the 5am basal rate needs to go down, because insulin peaks about two hours after its initial delivery into the body. This is just a quick glimpse into a Type 1's life and all of the thought and care that goes into making sure everything on the pump runs smoothly. It is definitely hard and time-consuming but it is something that, as Type 1 diabetics, we have to do. It's just another part of the deal. And to think we do all of this just to see the sun rise!

Okay, now that you know about all of the intricacies of my daily life, I think we can finally get into the more exciting things. But before I tell you about my struggles and accomplishments with T1D (oh yeah duh, T1D is an abbreviation for Type 1 diabetes because yes, I am that lazy), I think you should probably know what came before it....

The Good Old Days

I was born on February 7, 2001 in Northern Westchester Hospital in New York. I lived a normal childhood for the most part. I was born a chubby, happy baby so all was great in my parents' eyes. Three months before my third birthday, my sister, Caroline was born and when I was six, my brother Luke was born. Needless to say, it was a busy household.

Once my siblings were old enough to have any sort of opinion that differed from my own, the usual sibling rivalries and arguments began. The classic one that went on in my house was when I would be upstairs doing homework and Luke would be downstairs yelling, "Morgan pushed me off of the couch!" All of that sort of crap. And magically it was always my fault. You know how it goes, the oldest is always blamed and the youngest is the golden child. Trust me, it doesn't change.

When I was young, my parents put me in every sport you could imagine: soccer, lacrosse, dance, and softball (I'm not exactly graceful...we'll just say that in regard to why dance didn't work out). I had been there, done that. I hated every single one except lacrosse.

When I was thirteen I tried to explain my experience in lacrosse, *I liked lacrosse. So in kindergarten, I started playing. I was awful. But as the years went on, I progressed. In fifth grade, I shockingly made the A team in lacrosse (back then we called it the black team to not hurt anyone's feelings). Anyways, I played on the black team and surprisingly, you didn't want to cover your eyes every time I had the ball in my stick unlike my first few years with a stick in my hand. When I was six, I had started riding horses but never thought it would turn into anything. I thought it would just be a hobby.*

In sixth grade, I decided I didn't want to play anymore; I wanted to focus on horseback riding full time. It took some major convincing. I begged for weeks and at first it seemed like my mom wasn't going to budge since she played lacrosse for the University of Lynchburg in Virginia, but eventually she agreed. To this day she'll tell you that she made a mistake with the first one; don't let your child focus on one sport in sixth grade. But I did. I rode four or five days per week and the more I rode the better I became. Eventually, I was riding six days a week and showing competitively, until my uphill battle came.

The Berrie Center

The day after my pediatrician called and flipped my entire world upside down, my aunt came over bright and early to watch my siblings so my mom and dad could take me to New York City to see what my new life really had in store. Eye-opening is probably the best word to describe it. We spent the whole day at Naomi Berrie. I remember driving in the car on the way into the city. I had no idea, that I would no longer be "a normal kid."

I will never forget sitting in the backseat of our car saying to my parents, "It's okay, as long as I don't need blood work or a shot." Although my mom knew this was exactly what was going to happen to me several times per day for the rest of my life, she didn't want to scare me. It was every six-year-old's nightmare, needles. Little did I know when I made that comment, that I was going to be getting my finger pricked fifteen times per day, and being injected with insulin every time I ate, every time my blood sugar was high, and an additional shot for basal, for the rest of my life.

At the Berrie Center, we got a crash course on how to

deal with T1D, what to prevent, and what to do in different situations. During the crash course, we learned to avoid (as much as possible) high and low blood sugars, both of which are fatal if not treated quickly and properly. This sounds great in theory, just avoid highs and lows. But trust me when I say it is way easier said than done. The problem with this theory is that in many cases, highs and lows are unavoidable.

Before we continue, I want to give you a heads up that from here on I am going to include portions from an older version of my book that I wrote when I was between the ages of twelve and fifteen. This portion reads more like a journal. The excerpts taken from my journal will be in italics.

We got home late that night so I went straight to bed. Sure enough a few hours later, my blood sugar was high and I needed a shot. I still remember to this day, kicking and screaming in the bathroom at two in the morning because my dad told me I needed a shot. I was screaming bloody murder. It was one of those things that you remember so clearly because it was so scarring. That was possibly one of the worst nights of my life.

Being a frustrated and stubborn six-year-old, I was not going to have that damn shot whether it come hell or high water. So, let's leave it at this: it was a rough night for us all, and I'm pretty sure none of us (especially my parents who were scared out of their minds) got much sleep. I mean you can't blame them; their oldest child was just diagnosed with a life-threatening disease and here they were, having to give their child a drug that was necessary, but potentially fatal at the same time. Talk about a lot of pressure. My life was in their hands. Literally.

I often think about the emotional impact all of this had on my parents. As I mentioned before, they were dosing a drug that could either save or kill me, but the part that I would imagine is worse, is the fact that as they were actively trying to keep me alive, they had to watch their child hate her life with every ounce of her body. If I were a parent, that part of it would beat me up the most. I truly don't know how they did it.

We took it one day at a time as a family. It was difficult, but eventually we got through the weekend. Looking back today, I was very lucky because most people end up in the hospital, some even in a coma and that's how they find out that they have T1D. I am so thankful that I had my mom, who was already aware of the symptoms, to save me from that trip to the hospital; and maybe even my life.

But the most important thing I took away from this challenging time in my life was that when you are overwhelmed, you can't sit there and feel bad for yourself. Some things in life just suck, and those things you unfortunately cannot change. But I learned that when you hit those rough patches, you have to look ahead instead of throwing a pity party. Try to think about all of the opportunities that whatever tragedy you're going through is going to bring, because there will be something positive that comes out of it. There always is. In my case, that positive outcome is giving me the opportunity to communicate with you right now, and to share my story. I am hopeful that my story will inspire others going through hard times, and let them realize that although things might not get easier, they are going to be okay.

Family

For me, family is the top priority in life. I have a ton of aunts, uncles, and cousins, so my parents were constantly trying to instill the importance of family into our lives. "Friends come and go, but family…they are the ones who stay," my dad would say. And I full-heartedly believe him.

The dynamic in my household is different than most. We often joke that if a stranger were to walk in at any given point we would all be committed to some sort of mental institution. For starters, there is a significant amount of explicit language that is used by all family members at any moment in time. The tables have definitely turned considering I didn't know the word "shit" until seventh grade and I'm pretty sure Luke learned it at three years old. I guess they gave up trying to hide curse words from the third child.

My parents are constantly joking with us, but I'm not talking about joking in the traditional sense. It's more of sarcastic bullying if you ask me. First there's my mom who mocks just about everything I say, and then my dad who is constantly informing me of how much he "strongly dislikes" (the word "hate" is forbidden so the substitute is generally "strongly dislike" which is ironic considering all of the other horrible words we use) the bun I wear when my hair is either not cooperating, or desperately needs to be washed. Oh and how could I forget…on a daily basis, my mom tells me that I'm "too chatty." I try to explain to her that most people my age want nothing to do with their parents, and she should be thankful for how talkative I am but she doesn't usually buy it. Before I go further, you should probably know that although I'm making them sound like terrible people here, every single "insult" that comes out of one of my family members' mouths is out of pure love and humor.

Another running joke is that all we eat for dinner is either soup or chicken. My mom makes about twenty trillion different chicken dishes and I'm convinced, just rotates them day to day. Occasionally she'll throw in a night where we order pizza or Chinese food to make it seem like she's changing it up a bit, but she certainly hasn't fooled me.

Caroline and Luke don't get as "bullied" as I do. Probably because Luke is too sensitive and cries when you tell him he needs to brush his hair (or he used to at least), and Caroline is either never home or when she is, she's doing her own thing. She's out a lot playing either soccer or lacrosse depending on the season, but when she's home her eyes are glued to her computer where she binge-watches Netflix all day long. So that leaves me to take the brunt of my parents' sarcastic bullying when I'm not at the barn.

I often think about the way my parents raised my siblings and me. I adore the way that they are constantly poking fun and joking around. It definitely gave me thicker skin and the sense of humor I have today. But it isn't just my personality that my parents are responsible for. They keep me centered. They are the ones who support me day in and day out. They are willing to listen when I want to bitch about how awful my day was, and how I feel like crap because my damn infusion site has an air bubble. They are willing to leave me alone when I'm frustrated and just need to cry in the shower. They are willing to do all of this and everything in between. It is so important to have a strong support system behind you, especially when dealing with something difficult. If I didn't have their love, sense of humor, and encouragement every step of the way, I wouldn't be able to fight the battles against my body every single day. These battles are a part of the war that I call my life.

Yet Another Thing

As if Type 1 wasn't enough, in 2013 when I was twelve years old, I was diagnosed with hypothyroidism. This is a disease where your thyroid gland does not produce enough thyroid hormone (now that I'm reading that back it sounds really stupid and like such a basic definition but that's what it is). If untreated, an individual's metabolism, body temperature, and heart rate can be affected. My diagnosis came from some abnormal blood work results.

The treatment for this disease is much simpler than that of Type 1; it is just a pill at the same time every morning, generally prior to breakfast (which I don't usually eat anyway). But before my dosing became more consistent, we had to play a little game of trial and error. I tried a few different doses until we found the correct one. I stayed on that original dose for a while, but as I grew we discovered that my dosing needed to increase. We did another round of trial and error, which brought me to the dose I am on today. I continue to monitor my hypothyroidism via blood work that my endocrinologist orders once per year.

Although it doesn't demand the tireless thought and strain on my body that Type 1 does, having hypothyroidism just adds one more thing to my plate. It is a pain to have to remember to take a pill but if I could pick just one of these diseases to live with, it would without a doubt be hypothyroidism. Relative to everything else I have to deal with, taking a pill seems like nothing.

School

The Monday following my diagnosis, I had to go back to school. Both petrified and excited to get back to my routine, I went to the nurse's office with my parents to learn the ropes of what would happen while I spent time out of the comfort of my own home. The nurse, Mrs. Greenwood, was absolutely incredible. She took my parents and me under her wing, and from the first day I walked into school with Type 1 in Kindergarten until the day I graduated fifth grade, she could not have been more supportive. She was a crucial part to my success in school (and ultimately not dying all through elementary school).

Our kindergarten was only half-day so I went to after school enrichment which was three days a week and a whole other story. There was no nurse there so my dedicated and patient mom met me off the bus at enrichment every day I had it. She came to give me a shot in order for me to be able to eat lunch. I was so lucky I had her. I can honestly say, I don't know what I would do without her. She is not only my mom but my best friend. I laugh every time I am around her. Sorry that was off topic but she really is incredible!

Looking back on my time at middle and high school, I am so thankful for all of the staff who were always so supportive of me. I truly would not have been able to succeed without them. Each and every teacher I had has helped me grow and has touched my life in one way or another. I have learned so much, not only about science and math, but about myself through my teachers at school.

It is so important to constantly be trying to increase your knowledge and improve upon what you already know. Not to be the smartest one in your math or history class, but because it allows you to grow on a personal level. You learn things about yourself that you normally never would have, and the better you know yourself, the better you can understand how to improve your attitude. It is those with the best attitude who enjoy life the most, and have the easiest time achieving greatness.

Riding and Sports

As I mentioned prior, when I was around five or six I tried every sport you can imagine and cried in all of them. When I reached seven years old in first grade, I finally found something I enjoyed. Well I'm not sure I enjoyed it, it was more like I didn't cry every time I went so my parents assumed I was having a good time. From first through fifth grade, I played lacrosse.

As I started to get older, managing the low blood sugars as I was constantly running was difficult. I became frustrated that this disease was limiting me from playing at my full capacity. Every time I would get on the field and play hard for five minutes, I had to come off because I was low. It started becoming a cycle that I couldn't break. The fact that this miserable disease was getting the best of me was infuriating. Don't get me wrong, there are tons of people who successfully play a game of trial and error to determine the right combination of insulin and carbs for them to be able to continue playing the sport they love, but I didn't love lacrosse enough to do that. It's also tough because it's not like one size fits all in regard to a combination of carbs and insulin. Type 1 is a very individualized disease which is why we have to play the trial and error game. After a lot of time debating, I ultimately decided to stop playing after fifth grade. I don't want to say that the main reason I quit was because of Type 1 because it wasn't, but it did definitely make my decision a little bit easier.

I had been interested in horses all of my life. I first rode a horse at a fair when I was one year old! My dad will tell you that was the biggest mistake of his life, letting me ride a horse. He always tells me if I quit riding and go back to lacrosse he'll buy me a lacrosse stick made of gold because nothing will make up for the cost of riding. I began riding at my pediatrician's house because she lived on a farm. Her daughter, Emmy, trained me for four years. She was awesome! Then when I was ten, I moved to Rhiannon Equestrian.

I slowly got more and more into riding as I got older. I had been riding all along since I was six, but instead of only riding two days per week like I had been doing for the previous years, I decided to ride four days a week, then five, then six. Eventually I decided that this is what I love to do and by riding, Type 1 couldn't and wouldn't limit me (most of the time).

I am still an avid rider. I absolutely love riding. It puts me in a whole other world. Being with another living thing that doesn't speak makes it an extremely difficult and skill-based sport. We must figure out a way to communicate with these animals through body language (squeezing both legs, just your outside leg, half-halting on the reins, stuff like that). It forces you to be one hundred percent focused all of the time. And the part that bugs me the most is that people think it is just so easy; they think the horse does all of the work. Horseback riding takes an incredible amount of skill and strength. You must tell the horse where you want it to leave the ground from when you are jumping. And, you can get really hurt and even die doing it. It is not the safest sport and no, it is definitely not easy. But that is the part I love about it. Just like any other sport, you must work to get better, and practice does pay off.

All throughout middle and high school I rode six days a week. Whenever my school friends asked if I was free to hang out any day except Monday (when the barn is closed) they knew the answer would be, "No I have to ride." Riding takes up a huge part of my time, but I allow it to because I love it so much. I have formed such an amazing bond with Gideon over the years. I ride him (and give him treats of course) as much as I can, but it's difficult now that I'm in college. In case you were wondering, his favorite treats are bananas, Nature Valley honey and oats granola bars, and Welch's fruit snacks. He became a Welch's fan because that is my snack when my blood sugar is low. I usually eat a pack as I'm walking up to the ring which generally keeps me stable over the course of my ride. I'm not the biggest fan of the peaches gummies that come in the pack so Gideon gets those. He's mastered the skill of putting his head on my shoulder and nudging me until I feed him. There I go getting side-tracked again; sorry about that! Anyway, in the summer I bathe him after I ride and in the winter I put on his blankets (yes, he wears blankets). He's actually pretty funny—he knows how to unzip my jacket! When I am petting him, he will just come up and lick my face, too. (But I'm not going to lie; it's kind of gross when he licks my face). Gideon and I really do appreciate each other so much. Without an animal to love and care for, I would be lost.

I am so thankful that I have been fortunate enough to ride horses. It is, without a doubt, the biggest thing that keeps me going in my day-to-day life. Riding is one of the only types of exercise and sports where I don't feel limited by Type 1. But it didn't happen overnight. As I mentioned prior, I had to do a lot of trial and error that eventually led me to cutting back my basal rates two hours before I ride.

It occurs to me now that one of the main reasons I love riding so much is because it gives me somewhere to decompress. I need a place to go when I am feeling down on myself and beaten down by my disease. The barn gives me somewhere to forget everything, let go of all of my frustrations, and just ride. Often times when I've had a bad day and don't feel up to riding, I will still go to the barn anyway to be with Gideon. There is something inexplicable about the way he interacts with me, and it always puts me in a better, happier mood. Everyone needs a place that comforts them the way the barn comforts me.

I would like to thank my parents for supporting me through everything and allowing me to have this incredible opportunity because I truly do not think I could've gotten to where I am today without riding.

Faith

A huge part of why I never quit and never gave up was because of my faith. I am Roman Catholic and without God to pray to, I couldn't have gotten through all of the hard times. My family is more religious than most; we go to church every Sunday, and every night before we eat dinner, we pray as a family. It is so great to know that you have someone to go to when things aren't going your way. When something in my life is going wrong, I pray. Whether it's thanking God for what I have, asking Him to make my next day better, or praying the rosary; I know I can always look to Him and know He's there to help and guide me.

Before we go any further, I feel like I need to stop here and tell you something. Although I am speaking about my own connection to God and the impact He's had on my life, I am by no means trying to convince you that my viewpoint is the correct one, and I am not asking you to jump on board. I completely acknowledge that there are many different religions in this world and I respect every single one. I'm only telling you this because it has influenced my life in such a huge way that my story didn't feel complete without it. Just keep that in mind as you continue reading.

One thing I never understood about life in general is how bad things always happen to good people. (I am not AT ALL talking about me because trust me, if you know me well, I have a TON of flaws and am by no means "good!") One example of this is my grandfather. He passed away when I was just one year old. In 2002, he was on the auto train coming home from Florida because, ironically, he was scared to fly on a plane. The train derailed and he was one of four passengers to die on the train. I don't really remember him well because I was only one, but from what my mom, dad, and grandma tell me, he was an amazing man. On another note, my great uncle who was like a father figure to my dad passed away in 2015; he was a victim of brain cancer. He and my great aunt were as close as a couple could be; they did absolutely everything together (even going to the gym!). They are such generous and good-willed people. At only sixty-seven years old, it was so hard to watch him suffer and deteriorate so rapidly. I could never understand. Such good people, gone.

One day I just got so angry while I was in the shower. I know it's extremely strange and you're thinking, "This girl is bizarre - why does she ponder life and then get angry IN THE SHOWER of all places???" The shower is just where I think. I think about everything. I can focus really well there. (Before you read on, please realize that this is an incredibly bad sin that I'm about to admit to, but I have gone to confession since committing this terrible act so hopefully God forgives me). I got angry with God. I just didn't understand. It didn't make any sense why such bad things would happen to such good people. Then it hit me: the reason God takes such good people is because He wants them to be in a better place. I took this idea and applied it to people with chronic illnesses. My dad once told me that God gives bad diseases to people He thinks can handle them. But when he said this, I just kind of shook it off and did the "Whatever Dad, you're crazy" kind of teenage girl thing. But that day in the shower, I realized he was right. I started thinking about all of the people I know with Type 1 diabetes. And all of them are such strong, independent, and impressive people (Besides myself. I am an outlier for sure). From that day on, I realized that God isn't trying to harm anyone; He is trying to help them.

God plays such a key role in my everyday life. His teachings have not only shaped all of my morals and values, but they have helped me in times of crisis. Every night I pray. And at times of doubt when I am feeling down, I cannot imagine not having someone to go to. Without God in my life, there is no doubt I would not be the same person; probably a much worse one.

Again, please remember that I am not trying to convince you that my faith is the only one; I am simply telling you this because it is something that has helped me throughout the difficult times in my life.

Just recently I spent time thinking about the way God's act of giving me T1D shifted my perspective on life. I often see and hear people overreacting and getting upset over something that may seem big to them, but in reality is quite small. This is not necessarily that individual's fault; I do it, too. It is just that his/her life has not been put into perspective yet. Sometimes people need to experience some sort of tragedy in order for them to acknowledge how small the little things actually are. As difficult as that is, it is such an essential part of life. I am so thankful that God put my life into perspective for me at such a young age because it has enabled me to love it and enjoy every single moment that I stand here on this Earth.

If God hasn't put your life into perspective for you yet, do not wait for Him to do it; try to let the little things go, and only worry about the big ones. Those little ones do not deserve your time and energy.

Job Switch

As I said earlier, my dad was in real estate at the time of my diagnosis. He leased commercial office space in New York City. However, right after my great grandmother Leona Helmsley passed away in 2007, my dad was named one of the trustees of the Leona M. and Harry B. Helmsley Charitable Trust. It was hardly fate that my dad was named a trustee only a few months after I was diagnosed with Type 1.

He suddenly knew what his new mission in life was... improving the quality of life for people with Type 1 diabetes. My dad did what every other dad with a child in this situation would do; he quit his job in real estate and started working for the trust full time. It was difficult for him at first because he didn't know the first thing about Type 1 and philanthropy. He did quite a bit of research and traveling to meet with many different people to help him figure out what was in store for him with this new job.

He still works for the trust now and does a lot of traveling. Since he got this new job, he has also done a lot of public speaking. Just recently my mom and I were laughing because we called him to check in while he was away and he answered the phone by saying, "Hey, what's up? I'm about to go on stage." We found it humorous because if you know my dad at all, he does not seem like that serious guy who would be able to present to a group of people.

The amount my dad has accomplished over the years is incredible. To date, the trust has given over six hundred million dollars to Type 1 diabetes alone. That's unreal if you ask me. He is so amazing and I am so thankful that he took this route in life because he's perfect for a job like this. He continuously says that all he wants to do is help people dealing with this burden; he surely has done just that. I remember growing up, my dad would always tell me, "If I could trade places with you, I would do it in a second." If that isn't a caring and good-willed person, I don't know what is. To this day, his goal is to lighten the load and help people manage T1D. He continues to tell me and many others, "God laid this in my hands because this is my purpose in life: to help Morgan and all of the others dealing with this relentless disease."

Now sitting back and reflecting on this big coincidence, it hardly seems like one. It feels like this fell into my dad's lap not as a strange coincidence, but as an opportunity. An opportunity to help his daughter. An opportunity to change the world. There have been a bunch of instances in my life where I have felt like all of the puzzle pieces fell into place. I would spend countless days and nights worrying about one thing or another and how nothing in life would work out. But it honestly seems like magic when everything that originally seemed like your worst nightmare resolves itself. So in times when your life feels like it couldn't be any worse, try to remember that whatever is meant to be will always be.

On My Own

Six weeks after my diagnosis, I was fed up. I was fed up with the fact that I had T1D. I was fed up with my parents for making me do these stupid shots (of course they were only trying to keep me alive but what did I know at six years old?). I was fed up with my life. All I kept wondering as an innocent little six-year-old was, *Why me? Why did it have to be me?* And my mom would tell me every day, "You are in this situation because God knows you're strong enough to be in it. He doesn't give this life to just anyone. Only the ones he knows have the strength to handle it." Well every time my mom would tell me this, it set a fire in me (and no, not to the rain, either. Sorry, I'm kind of obsessed with Adele). Anyway, I decided that if I have the strength to deal with this disease, I should be able to deal with it all by myself. So one day when my blood sugar was high and I needed a shot, my dad was going to give it to me. I remember saying to him, "No! I want to do it!" He replied, "Okay sure, go for it."

I sat in my little monogrammed pottery barn pink chair that was big enough to fit a pea, and I held the syringe in my hand. I could tell you exactly what room I was sitting in. And that was two houses ago! I was not going to quit until I gave myself that stupid shot. I remember sitting in my chair crying. I was frustrated. I was annoyed. And most of all, I was determined to do this damn shot. After forty-five minutes of crying and trying to overcome the huge amount of fear I had in that moment, I did it. I gave myself a shot for the first time.

No words can describe what I was feeling at that moment: excitement, pride, power, to name a few. Probably most of all, the awe that I actually did it with no help at all. From then on, I didn't look back. There were no more shots from my parents. It was all me all of the time. I wonder if the reason it felt so good to be able to do my own shot is because it allowed me to release some of my emotions that had been bottled up for so long. Everyone has those things that they stuff under the bed because they don't want to let them out. Trust me, I have them too. But the reality is that not expressing your emotions is unhealthy; we need some sort of mechanism to cope with difficult times. At that moment when the needle punctured my skin, the stress and anger that had been building up all along was released. This was my way of coping with the fact that my life had been flipped upside down just six weeks earlier, and it felt so good.

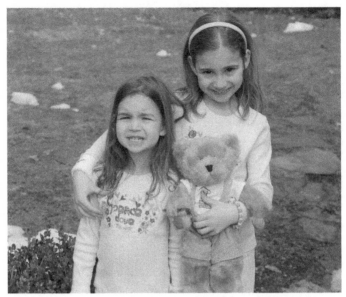

Caroline and I the day after I was diagnosed with my diabetic bear named Rufus. Prior to my diagnosis I lost 11 pounds which is why my face looks so thin. That's a lot of weight for a six year old!

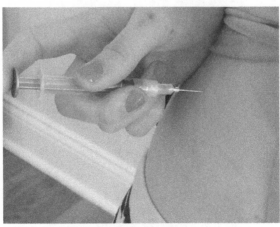

One of the daily insulin injections I had to do. Most days it was between eight and twelve shots per day before I got my pump.

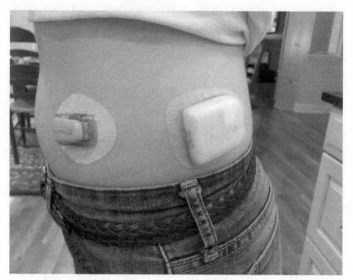

Both my CGM (left) and pod (right) so you can get a sense of what they look like.

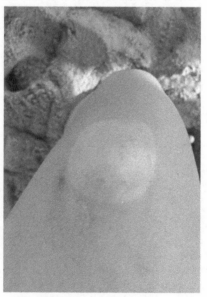

One of the many perks of the summer…pod tans!

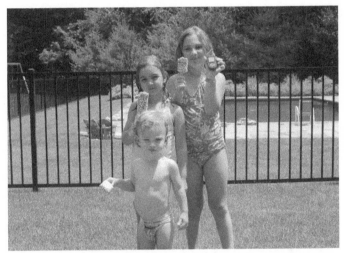

Luke, Caroline, and I eating a chocolate eclair after a nice swim in the pool! I was seven, Caroline was four, and Luke about a year. For some reason I seem very excited to hold up my pump for the camera...

Part II

"No matter how much it hurts now, one day you will look back and realize it changed your life for the better."

ANONYMOUS

One Foot in Front of the Other

After three months of getting a feel for Type 1 and being on shots, my endocrinologist allowed me to get an insulin pump. My mom recently told me that the day I got my pump I looked at my parents and said, "This is the happiest day of my life." My mom said she remembers thinking about how sad it was that the happiest moment of her six-year-old's life was getting an insulin pump. Although in all fairness, being able to eliminate eight to twelve shots every day was a complete game-changer. Shots (and needles overall) are every child's nightmare, so the fact that I could now wear an insulin pump with a tube connecting to an insertion on my body instead of shots was amazing. The only catch was that I had to change the insertion location in my body every other day. But remembering the multiple shots per day, changing my pump site felt like a breeze. There is no doubt that this disease sucks from every angle you look at it, but the first day of using my pump was possibly the best yet in 2007.

My mom, dad, and I once again spent the day at Naomi Berrie Diabetes Center learning the ins and outs of this new device. After the first week of using just saline, (almost like water so that if I overdosed by accident, it wouldn't kill me like insulin would) we went back to Columbia one more time. Finally they switched the saline out for insulin, and I was wearing a full-fledged insulin pump. I was thrilled!

At first when I wore it, I felt like an alien. Walking around school with a fanny pack and tubing coming out of it leading to my body was a little weird. Especially for a little kindergartener. But soon enough I realized that in order to stay alive this was going to be how it is, and I was going to have to deal with it.

The only down side to the pump was that because there was a tube coming out of it, it would get stuck in my locker or on the swings and rip out. Then my mom would have to come to school and bring supplies for me to do a new one. It was a production, but still significantly better than the alternative.

The pump is very difficult for anyone, especially a six-year-old, to use and navigate. It is also a huge responsibility because if I gave myself too much insulin, I could die. It was a ton of weight to carry on my shoulders, and a little frightening, too.

During school I had to go to the nurse about three or four times a day on a strict schedule: before snack, before lunch, before I got on the bus to go home, before and after gym class (physical activity makes your blood sugar go low, but I'll get into that more later), and then anytime I was high or low. The reason for this was basically to make sure I wasn't going to go low while on the bus going home, and making sure I put in the correct number of carbs into my pump before lunch or snack.

Prior to using an insulin pump, my life felt like a true nightmare. This entire concept of getting my first pump may seem like something small to you, but for me it was a milestone. It was the marker of the first mile. Once I hit that very first marker, I felt a sense of accomplishment. It was comforting to think that if I had been able to get through the days in the beginning with only a bunch of syringes and test strips, I would certainly be able to run the rest of this damn marathon with the development of technology. It is incredible to see how all of the technology has evolved over the years. Once I got my pump, I couldn't imagine life without it, and now that I have my CGM, I can't even begin to wonder how different my life would be if I was not fortunate enough to have it. But at the end of the day, always remember that sometimes in life you can't take that initial leap of faith so soon. You have to take a couple of baby steps forward before you have the ability to make the jump.

Walk 4 Morgan

A year after I was diagnosed, my parents first heard about how people do "walks." At these walks, you invite pretty much everyone you know and they come to walk with you in honor of Type 1 diabetes. The goal is to raise money for an organization called the Juvenile Diabetes Research Foundation, more commonly known as JDRF. After doing some research, my parents found one that had been taking place at the Bronx Zoo in years past, and shortly after they decided to sign me up. We created a team called, "Walk 4 Morgan."

"Walk 4 Morgan" consisted of almost everyone I knew. From family to friends, people my dad worked with, teachers, school nurses, and everyone in between, they all came to support me. As a young kid, I remember being so excited every year prior to the walk to see the animals with all of my friends and family. My family and I designed new T-shirts every year and when they were delivered, I would separate them all by size. My next job was to label them with everyone's names and what size they asked for. It was so much fun! The night before the

walk, I would stay up really late unable to fall asleep because I was so excited for the day to follow.

The next morning, my family would get up way too early, pack the car, and off we went to the zoo. When we got there, I would set up our table and our sign labeled "Walk 4 Morgan" in elaborate letters, and get everything ready for when my friends and family arrived. When they came, I would give them their T-shirt and wrist band. We then walked around the zoo admiring all of the animals. I used to look forward to that day all year. My T-shirt even won first place in the T-shirt contest one year! Unfortunately after a few years, the Bronx Zoo stopped hosting it and that was the end of "Walk 4 Morgan."

Now thinking back, I think the reason I was so passionate and excited for the walks was because it was a day for my peers to acknowledge what I went (and go) through. To say that being at war with your body three hundred and sixty-five days per year for twenty-four hours per day is hard, is an understatement. As a young child I would get frustrated that people didn't really think about how much thought I had to put into eating an apple, for example; a simple task that requires zero thought for every other person on the planet except for me (or so I thought). The days that everyone walked for me when I was younger gave me reassurance that people were conscious of what I go through, and they were trying to understand. To me, the fact that they were even attempting to understand, meant the world.

Children's Congress

In 2009 when I was eight years old, I got an incredible opportunity. I was able to go to Washington D.C. to an event called Children's Congress hosted by the Juvenile Diabetes Research Foundation (JDRF), with ninety-nine other Type 1 diabetics. They chose two children from each state to serve as delegates, meet their state's senators, and tell their story in order to lobby Congress for more funding for T1D.

After I applied and was accepted to the event, my family worked out our travel plans. My dad and I caught a plane on a Wednesday morning and headed down to Washington D.C., while my mom and Caroline came the next day. Luke was still young so he stayed home with my grandma, Mimi.

The first thing I remember after arriving, was going into a huge room in the hotel and meeting all of the other kids with Type 1 who were also chosen as delegates. It was the first time I actually realized that I wasn't the only one with this disease. There were people of all ages that had it, too. Then, a woman came in to address the group. She said that we were going to take a field trip. A field trip? I thought. Sounds fun! First we went to meet the senators from New York. At the time, they were Kirsten Gillibrand and John Hall. After a few hours with them, we then proceeded to the White House. Yes, we went to the White House, and yes we met the president at that time, Barack Obama. Now that, was cool. I remember all of us sitting on the steps in front of the White House and there was this little boy, probably four or five years old running around crying. President Obama got up off the steps and said, "Come here little guy," picked him up, and plopped him right on his lap. That's where he stayed for our group picture. We were all squinting in the picture, too, because man was it sunny!

After meeting the president, my dad and I returned to the hotel room. I was looking forward to relaxing for the remainder of the day. It had been exhausting for my little eight-year-old legs. Then, my dad said, "Morgan you only have thirty minutes. Then we are going to leave again." I tried to tell him that I was exhausted and wasn't moving, but it was a good thing he made me get off of my lazy butt because turns out we were going to meet some more amazing people. First, we had a private meeting with Nick Jonas, a fellow Type 1 diabetic.

After meeting Nick, we returned to the whole group and hung out with Jared Allen, an NFL football player (who was on the Minnesota Vikings at the time), and Sugar Ray Leonard (a former professional boxer). I think my dad might have been more excited to meet them than I was. What did I know about football and boxing as an eight-year-old girl?

When I was at the event back in 2009, I knew it was a great opportunity but I didn't truly understand the real reason I was there. At the time I thought I was there to meet Obama and to see that I wasn't alone in my journey. But I now know that it was so much more than that. I was there to fight for the pricy drug that keeps me alive. I was trying to show legislators the importance of insurance companies covering my supplies. This is a reoccurring issue that affects my family every single day. I do not understand how this is even a question, to be honest with you. I'm not exactly asking for them to cover some unnecessary cosmetic procedure, just the drug that saves my life.

I cannot begin to tell you the amount of time my dad spends on the phone fighting with our insurance company. Although they do cover one generic type of insulin, this type in particular did not work for me. I would spend entire days on the couch throwing up because my blood sugar was over 350mg/dL and still, our insurance company refused to cover any other type of insulin. More recently, after getting a letter from my doctor explaining the issue along with evidence from my CGM of the days I spent at unhealthily high glucose levels, they decided they would cover it after rejecting our plea the first three times. But this battle is still being fought by people every day. I am honored that I was able to help the fight, and I hope in the future I will be able to continue to make a difference not for me, but for all of the other people out there who are going through the same hell that I did.

First There Was One, and Then There Were Two

The years following my diagnosis were the toughest. There were no words to describe the journey. Between the amount of tears, needles, and pump failures, more than anything else it made me realize that I would not wish this disease on anyone; especially my own family. However, it seemed it was already on the way for Caroline.

A year after finding out I had Type 1, my parents decided it would be a good idea to have my siblings screened to see if they had any of the antibodies, considering genetics is thought to possibly play a role in the victims of T1D. After going for blood work, we came to the conclusion that Luke had zero of the four antibodies while Caroline had two out of the four. The doctor's response to this was, "It's fine, we will just keep an eye on it." But after six months things weren't looking too promising. Caroline had developed all four out of four antibodies. This brought us to the conclusion that she would get T1D too; it was just a matter of time.

Luckily, the government funded a clinical trial for family members of people with T1D, specifically for people like Caroline who had four out of four antibodies. The way it worked was half of the patients were given a placebo and the other half were given an oral insulin, in hopes of slowing the process down. Just recently we found out that Caroline had been on the placebo.

What this clinical trial consisted of was Caroline going to Columbia every six months for an OGTT, or in normal people terms, an oral glucose tolerance test. Basically she would drink this gross sugar-laden drink and sit in a chair with an IV for two hours. Then, the nurse would come in every twenty minutes to test her blood sugar. A few weeks after the test, my parents would get the results as to how fast T1D was developing for Caroline since it varies from individual to individual.

Unfortunately in July of 2017, Caroline was officially diagnosed with Type 1. She has started on a pump and loves to brag that hers is more "high-tech" than mine. Although I would never wish Type 1 on anyone, especially my own sister, I feel like there is no family more equipped to handle two kids with this disease than my own, simply because of how involved my parents have become.

Just recently I thought about the role Caroline's diagnosis has played in my own life. First of all, it taught me leadership. As you can imagine, it was hard for her to adjust (as it would be for anyone), mainly because she is an anxious person. Just like me, she hates change, a characteristic that we definitely inherited from my dad. At this crucial time in Caroline's life, I had to step up to the plate. My mindset had completely shifted. I was no longer fighting the fight for me, I was fighting for Caroline. I needed to show her that you can't let this shitty disease beat you down. It's not worth it.

Caroline is slowly learning to accept this new way of life. In hindsight it was both a blessing and a curse that I got Type 1 when I did. It was a blessing because I was so young that it's hard to remember life without it; this life is the only one I've ever known. But Caroline, who was diagnosed at age thirteen, can recall everything about her "old life" which makes it harder. I am beyond frustrated that God chose my sister as yet another victim but at the same time, I have to remember my faith. There is a reason that He chose her; she is strong, and she has an enormous support system of friends and family behind her.

Camp

Going into first grade, I went to a summer camp close to home. It was centered around a lake, which was where we would go swimming every day. The first year that I went after being diagnosed was, well, interesting to say the least.

The counselors and director were all very supportive; however, it was hard looking different from the other kids since we walked around in bathing suits all day. If I was older, I would have said, "Whatever, I'll get over it," but since I was only seven at this point and everyone would whisper and stare at me, it was hard. I didn't know what to do or what to say. So instead I said nothing, and it continued. But as I got older, I learned to talk to people and ask them if they have any questions. Not in a malicious way, but I figured that if I answered their questions, it might alleviate all of the staring, whispering, and pointing. Plus, it is good to get our country educated as this is a growing disease, and the majority of the U.S. is clueless (I know it seems harsh but it is the reality. Another thing you will learn about me if you haven't already is that I don't sugarcoat anything. Ever).

But swimming was a whole other battle. So, basically what you have to do with the tubing pumps is whenever you are going to take a shower, go swimming, etc., you have to disconnect the pump from your body since it's not waterproof. But the little insertion with the needle stays in your body. By disconnecting, all you are eliminating is the pump itself and the tubing. However, when I wasn't getting insulin while swimming, my blood sugar would go high. And then I got migraines and it was just a big mess. It was frustrating because at seven years old, I wasn't able to just be a kid and swim carefree like everyone else. I always had to think about my condition. I don't remember a time when I didn't have it on my mind.

Another difficulty was the insertion itself. Occasionally I would leave the water at free swim in camp to give myself a little insulin so I wouldn't go high, but when I got out of the water to do that, I would notice that the insertion that was supposed to be there, wasn't. What would happen was the adhesive would get weak and fall off from swimming so much. Then I would have to do a whole new insertion, which sucked, because I would have to stop swimming and having fun with my friends just to do a new site. It didn't seem fair that all of these other kids could swim for as long as they wanted without having to worry about their health, but I had to get out and manage my blood sugars.

Camp was hard because it was my first real encounter dealing with the public. I had to find a way to navigate looking and being different from everyone around me. The amount of people, especially adults, who would stare was unimaginable. You would have thought I was an alien with three heads! I wonder if dealing with this situation is the reason I have become so understanding of others who look different as well.

Martha

Let me start this off by saying that my mom is a dedicated runner. She will run in rain, snow, sub-zero temperatures, or one hundred degrees. She doesn't care. It's a running joke (pardon the pun) in our house because we call her Forrest Gump.

When I was diagnosed and my dad became involved with Type 1, aside from my daily care, my mom also wanted to make a difference. She began turning her passion of running into running races to raise money for T1D. My mom has run the New York City Marathon four times with Team JDRF in addition to numerous half marathons raising tens of thousands of dollars. She still runs the New York City Half Marathon every year with team JDRF and to date, she has raised over forty-five thousand dollars.

Anyway, one day she came home from her morning run and said, "Guys! You'll never believe who I just saw on her horse while I was running today. Martha Stewart! She wants Morgan and me to be on her show." We were in shock that my mom actually saw her. I don't know why, considering we live ten minutes away from her but whatever, that's beside the point.

My dad asked, "Are you gonna do it?"

"Of course!" my mom replied. The next thing I knew, a few weeks later when I was just a second grader, my mom said, "Alright Morgan, put a dress on, we are going to film a TV show!"

"What?"

"Just do it, would you? We're leaving in twenty minutes!"

"Okay," I replied. I put my little red dress on, a bow in my hair, and we were off.

My mom and I drove into New York City with one of my dad's work partners, Dana Ball, and we all went together. My dad stayed home with my brother and sister since all three of them had the flu.

When we got to the studio, they kindly invited us to sit in a room with all of Martha's Emmy awards. Real live Emmys. Dana and my mom were taking pictures of themselves holding one up and acting like they just won. It was hilarious! Then, a lady came in to put our microphones on and brought us to the set. We sat down and when they were ready to start shooting, Martha introduced us on the show.

It was a little nerve racking; I'm pretty sure I almost threw up before speaking but I didn't, so it was okay (if you can't tell, I'm petrified of public speaking. Well, I used to be. I've had to get used to it. You'll see what I mean later, but for now just keep reading). Then they started asking me questions: "How often do you check your blood sugar? What is the hardest part

about living with T1D? What do kids at school think of it?"
Those kinds of things. After I nervously answered their questions
as fast as I possibly could, they went to my mom.

Martha asked her about how she found out I had Type 1
and my mom shared my family's story. She answered the
questions in a poised manner and held herself together nicely.
Oh wait. Then she started tearing up on set which is completely understandable since it was, and always will be a
sensitive subject. The point is, it was a really great experience
for both of us and we still to this day joke about my mom
crying on camera (or as she likes to call it, "tearing up").

I went back to school the day after it aired, and my prin-
cipal decided to show it to the whole school. That was
objectively one of the most embarrassing moments of my
life. I'm pretty sure my face was beet red on the screen. Except
I wouldn't really know, because I didn't watch it. I stared at
the wall the whole time waiting for it to be over because I
was so damn embarrassed.

Filming with Martha was not only an amazing experience, but it marked the beginning of my advocacy in the
world of Type 1. By traveling into New York City and speaking
on Martha's show, I started to believe that as a young girl, I
had the ability to raise awareness and fight for myself and
others. I finally started to see that it didn't matter that I was
eight years old, or that I was just one person. The number of
us didn't matter; it was the passion. I guess what I'm trying
to say is, never think that one person is not enough to initiate
change. You can make up for the lack of numbers with your

drive and devotion. If you care enough and put your time in, you can change the world. You can do anything.

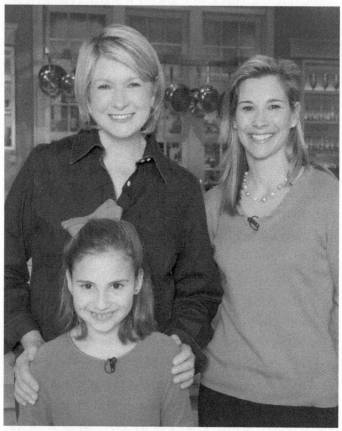

My mom and I snapped a quick picture after taping an episode on Martha Stewart's show.

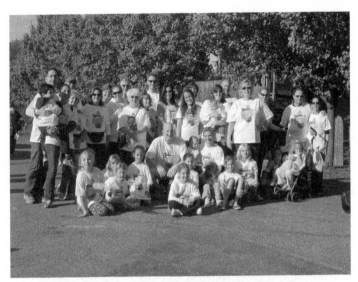

My "Walk 4 Morgan" team in 2007 held at the Bronx Zoo. It was my first walk ever! My family, friends, and even teachers came to my walks. This was one of our smaller teams since it was my first year doing it.

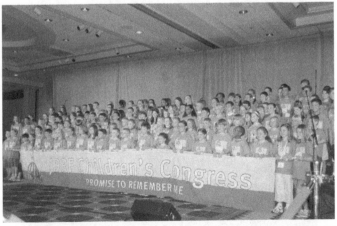

All of the Children's Congress 2009 delegates. Two Type 1 diabetic children from every state in the U.S. came to Washington D.C. I am the one standing on the floor holding up the sign (second from the end on the right).

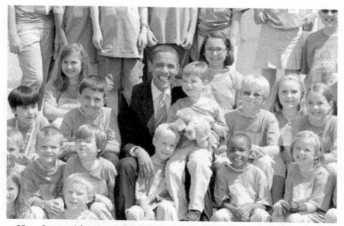

Here I am with some of the other kids from Children's Congress and President Obama. I am the one on the left next to him.

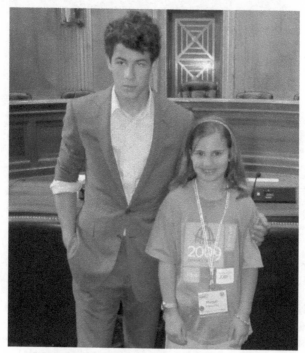

Nick Jonas and I at Children's Congress. I don't think he was as excited to meet me as I was him!

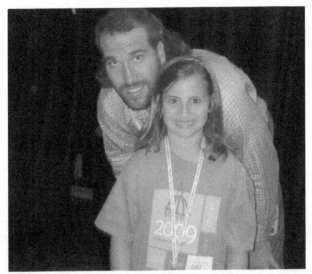

Here I am with NFL player Jared Allen.

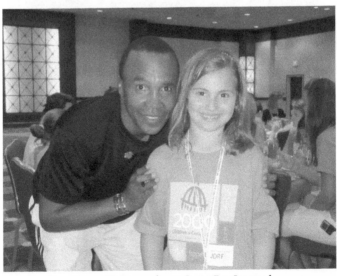

Here I am with famous boxer Sugar Ray Leonard.

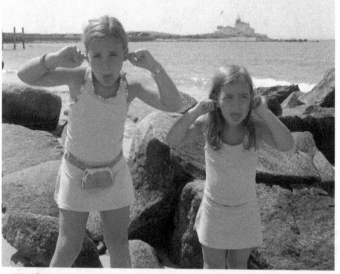

Here's Caroline and I in Nantucket one summer (we go every year).
As you can see, I had my pump pack on because this was when I used
the pump with the tubing (it was called the Cosmo).

Part III

"Whether you think you can or think
you can't you're right."

HENRY FORD

The Night from Hell, or Should I Say Heaven?

Having the job he does, my dad travels all over the world learning more about Type 1. He meets with the leading researchers and scientists that will help speed up making this disease more manageable. One night when I was in fifth grade and my dad was traveling, I was sleeping in my mom's room (when my dad was away, all of us would set up air mattresses in my parents' room and camp out. Don't ask, it was a tradition). It was around 8:30pm and I was getting ready to go to bed. I said, "Good night, Mom. I love you."

She replied, "Sweet dreams. Love you past the sky!"

At that moment, God himself must have sent a message straight down from Heaven telling my mom to test my blood sugar even though I had just tested half an hour before. If He hadn't, you wouldn't be reading this book right now because I wouldn't be here. So my mom decided to test me. She didn't really know why, but she did. My blood sugar was 54mg/dL. "Morgan, how are you 54? You just had dessert!"

"I have no idea!" I replied. I knew that this wasn't possible. I laid in bed just thinking. After two minutes, I said to my mom, "Wait a second…I had to change the battery of my pump, and I didn't disconnect the tubing when I primed it." Just in case you don't wear a pump or are not familiar with what this means, let me explain it to you.

My insulin pump runs on batteries, (yes, my pancreas is a AAA battery) and when you change the battery, you have to do something called priming the pump (side note: this only applies to the pumps with tubing, which is what I was wearing at the time). What this means is you have to disconnect the tubing from your body and watch the insulin come out to ensure the pump is working correctly and you will be getting insulin. However, I forgot to disconnect when I primed it. When my mom and I looked in the history of the pump, it said that I primed ten whole units of insulin into myself. To put things into perspective of how much this was for me at the time, I would have had to eat two large pizza pies to undo what was done…literally!

My mom was frantic, as I'm sure anyone would be if they weren't sure if they were going to see their child the next day. She immediately called my dad and told him what happened. She asked him if she should call 911. He told her absolutely not, their information hasn't been updated in years and in some instances, they don't even know what the current insulin types are. So my mom ran down the stairs as fast as her feet could carry her. She returned with a huge cup of orange juice filled to the top and ordered me to drink it.

As I started drinking it, I tasted clumps. "Ew what is this?" I asked her.

"Sugar. Now drink it, would you?" I drank three sixteen ounce cups of orange juice with three tablespoons of raw brown sugar in each one. Then I ate ten Swedish fish and was ready for bed.

"Good night, Mom," I said.

"No way!" she replied. "You can't go to bed."

"Why not?"

"Because I won't know if you are passing out from sleeping or being low. You have to stay awake until your blood sugar comes up." I laid in bed for an hour and a half, which at that point felt like years. I was so nauseous because of all of the food I had just consumed. It was one of those things where you think you'd feel better if you threw up, but I couldn't because if I did, I would have had to start all over again (drink the juice and eat the Swedish fish). Poor Caroline asked my mom, "Is Morgan going to die?" And the worst part was that my mom could not confidently say no.

Finally two hours later, my blood sugar came up but only to 74mg/dL. Not great, but at least it was heading in the right direction. I went to bed and thank God, woke up the next morning. I have never believed in God more. To this day, I truly believe it was Him who made my mom test me; and I will be eternally grateful for that.

I am now able to see that this experience was not only petrifying, but a wake-up call. It was the first time that I was able to wrap my head around the fact that this drug actually has the potential to kill me. That was especially frightening considering I was only ten years old, but it is important to keep things in perspective. It never hurts to be reminded every now and then as to how serious this disease is. Wake-up calls like this one keep me on my toes, and always remind me to double and triple check before hitting a button to deliver insulin. All it takes is the push of one button, to change everything.

Living Accommodations

Going into fourth grade, all of the sleepovers were beginning. As much as I wanted to go to my friends' houses and stay over, I was scared. The responsibility of having to take care of myself at night was daunting. I was happy having my friends over to my house, but the second it was at someone else's house, I was too nervous about what could happen. Even if my dad told me that he would pick me up at any time during the night, I wouldn't go.

I was afraid of being a burden to my friends' parents because if I did sleep over, my parents would have to wake them up in the middle of the night multiple times just because of me and my disease. Not to mention, just the idea of living alone in its entirety became increasingly concerning over the years as college approached.

I am living out all of my previous worries now that I am in college. It has been a huge adjustment from living at home with my parents, but I am starting to get the hang of it. A key reason for this fairly smooth transition is my roommate.

I met my college roommate through a friend I know from high school. The day after I got into Villanova, my friend came up to me and said "I know this girl Kirsten from CCD who is also going to Villanova, and I know you guys would get along really well." She gave me Kirsten's number, and I texted her a few weeks later. After talking the whole afternoon about pretty much everything, I realized I'd forgotten to ask her what her major is. My dad really wanted me to room with either a nursing or biology student because he figured they would understand more about Type 1. When she informed me she was a biology major hoping to go to medical school, I knew we would be a great match. I followed it up by asking what kind of doctor she wanted to be, and she responded with the following, "Well, I really like what both of my parents do, so maybe I could follow in their footsteps. My dad is a psychiatrist and my mom is an endocrinologist." What are the odds of that?

I went to dinner with Kirsten and her family a week later. We had a great time and after discussing our grandma-like sleeping habits, the fact that we aren't really partiers, and that we both want to continue going to church every Sunday at school, we realized that we were basically the same person. We even showed up to dinner wearing the same sweater. Talk about a freaky coincidence. Before we left the restaurant that night, we decided that we would make great roommates. I totally believe the entire situation was Divine intervention. (Side note: I made sure to tell Kirsten that I was going to drive her crazy beeping the whole night. She responded by saying, "Don't worry, I asked my mom to give me a T1D crash course before we get to school so I'll be prepared!")

Although I still worry about going to sleep and having to deal with this burden by myself at night with the possibility that I won't wake up, I am thrilled to know that I have a roommate who is willing to support me every step of the way. The truth is, this disease is frightening and it's scary. That's just the nature of it. But the only way to try and alleviate that fear is by making sure you're surrounded by people who are willing to help.

I'm not going to lie to you; it is frustrating having to set alarms every night to check my blood sugar. It doesn't seem fair that no one else has to go through this. But as I have gotten older, I've learned to put a positive spin on everything in life. Having to wake up to monitor my blood sugars has made me much more responsible, and will definitely benefit me in the long run.

Although I like to think that Type 1 can't limit me in any way, the truth is that it can sometimes. Sleepovers were tough when I was young, and living on my own is still tough for me now. This is annoying because it's something that is so mindless for everyone else. For most people, moving out and living on their own is something to look forward to, but for me it's a source of constant stress and anxiety.

Over the years I have learned to accept the fact that even though I don't want Type 1 to limit me and even though it's not fair, there are certain aspects of my life that are negatively impacted by my disease. There are things that are more difficult and require more thought than for my peers; and unfortunately, that is not something that I can change.

Frustration and Anger

There are so many instances where I am appalled by the ignorance of medical professionals. I don't know if they just don't care enough or if their education is outdated, but I have been offended and just simply annoyed with some of the things that people say.

To give you an example, there was one time when there was a bat in my house and we weren't sure if it had bitten or touched us, so my family and I had to go to the hospital to get rabies shots. After we finished (I had gotten four and three of them were in my butt so it was a traumatic experience) the nurse who administered the shots brought us ice pops. She went over to Caroline and Luke (this was before Caroline was diagnosed) and said, "Here would you guys like ice pops?" Then she looked at me and said, "Sorry you can't have any with your diabetes because these aren't sugar free." Wow. Just typing that was infuriating. I'm not sure who gave this individual her information, but it is one hundred percent incorrect. As I've said before, I can eat ANYTHING I want as long as I give myself insulin. Besides the fact that it is not acceptable to use the term "diabetes" anymore. It is really important to specify which type you're talking about because they are two completely different diseases.

Another occurrence where something like this happened was at the ophthalmologist. I was just getting a normal eye exam so the doctor had his assistant come in first to get my medical history. When I told him I had Type 1 he said the following, "Do you check your blood sugar at home?" I didn't mean to be rude, but when he said that I started laughing for no reason other than the fact that it was a ridiculous comment. I check my blood sugar fifteen times per day and if I didn't check it at home, I would have died a long time ago. Not sure who prompted this question, but not only is it completely useless, but it's ignorant. Again, I don't think these individuals did it to be malicious at all, I just think that their information is extremely outdated.

Because of experiences like these, part of what I want to do (besides being a pediatric endocrinologist) is travel the world educating people, especially medical professionals, to make them more informed of the severity of Type 1 diabetes. I want to teach them about what it is and what it means as far as daily life for all of those dealing with it. The least we can do is have people understand what we go through every freaking day!

Dealing with Emotions

One of the most significant struggles I've had while living with Type 1 is figuring out the right way to deal with my emotions. I am someone who keeps everything bottled up inside. I do not like to cry in front of anyone (although I've become increasingly soft as I get older), so instead I try my best to always keep up a strong face even when I'm distraught on the inside. This method has not proved to be worthwhile at all; rather, it often makes matters worse.

As I'm sure I've made abundantly clear by now, T1D is a physically exhausting disease, but I'm willing to argue that the emotional exhaustion is worse. Yes, I have scars all over my body from the countless finger pricks, pump infusion sets, and CGM sites, but nothing compares to how much thought goes into every single decision I make. I've learned to cope with the "normal" days, but I've found that the days where I get overly frustrated are the ones where my blood sugars are completely erratic. It's discouraging when I'm doing everything right and my body doesn't respond. There are times where I get home from school after having high or low blood sugars all day, and I just go to my room and cry because I don't know what to do. I've done everything I was taught and everything that I'm supposed to do. The fact that I see no results is upsetting; it makes me feel helpless. I'm trying my best to make it through the damn day and not only do I feel like shit, but nothing I do can fix it.

There was one day I remember, where I was at school and I asked my teacher to go to the bathroom. I locked myself in the stall and started crying. I couldn't hold it in anymore because my blood sugar had been so high the whole day. I had given myself over ten units of insulin and couldn't get below 300mg/dL. I remember just crying and crying for fifteen minutes because I didn't know what to do. I felt like it was such a low point in my life and I was stuck there. I couldn't escape; not for a day, not even for a minute.

The difficult part is, unlike other low points in one's life that you can momentarily try to forget about and revisit later, you can never wait and revisit Type 1. There isn't one second that I can try and forget about it because it's my life at stake. Don't get me wrong, there are certain days where I feel like a superhero because I'm kicking Type 1's ass, but there are many more days where I've hit rock bottom. It's frustrating because most people don't get it. They don't understand that there are some days where it may seem like I have everything under control. Those good days do exist, but they are few and far between. Then there are other days where nothing goes right. These days are much more frequent, and they are the ones where T1D is kicking the crap out of me. People can't see it, but I'm always fighting.

Over the years I've learned that the sucky days where you feel beaten down are the ones that make you stronger. But often times before you get stronger, you have to be weak. So don't be afraid to lie on the ground and sob your eyes out because you've done everything you can think of and nothing's going your way. It's acceptable to get mad and it's acceptable to cry. We're humans, we can't be superheroes all of the time. Let your emotions out, because when you come back from whatever you're going through, you're going to come back twice as strong if you let go of all the unnecessary baggage.

Friend Dynamic

Throughout my entire life, my friends (who are for the most part the same, you know who you are ladies) have been nothing but supportive of me. They are always trying to learn more about what I go through and they are always concerned when I am high or low.

I am so fortunate to have friends who never made fun of me, or made snarky comments; they have done nothing but cheer me on all the way. I am so glad that I'm able to say that T1D has not affected my friendship with this amazing group of girls.

My barn friends are amazing, too. We are one big family. Everyone there hears the beep of my CGM and is concerned. They all want to learn and want to help. When I run out of juice boxes, someone is willing to give me their food. When I am too low to ride, someone is willing to wait for me. I'll never forget this one time where I was riding Gideon and I was looking across the ring, and I could've sworn the fence was two inches away from my face. Meanwhile, it was entirely on the other side of the ring! So I figured it was probably time to get off. I hopped off of Gideon and tested my blood sugar. It was 27mg/dL! One of my friends who also rides at the barn, Leah, was in the tack room. The first thing I did was take a picture because that was a new record of how low I'd ever been. To give you an idea, some people have seizures and/or pass out at 45mg/dL. Leah said, "Morgan! What are you doing? You need a juice!" So she got me a juice and made me drink it.

It is so important to have a strong support system behind you. One of the main reasons that I have the power and strength to keep going is because I have people in my life who are not afraid to be in this with me. It makes me feel like this isn't my battle, it's our battle. A prime example of this are two of my friends from high school.

One day during our senior year, they came into school with a crazy idea. They thought it would be fun to see what it was like being a Type 1 diabetic. It sounded like a great idea to me, so they came over to my house the following weekend in what I would describe as a frenzy. The amount of questions that were being screamed at me was unbelievable. I cued up pumps and CGMs for the two of them to wear.

After an hour of practically begging them to go through with this and reminding them that it was their idea, I was finally able to get them to let me insert the CGM and pump infusion site. My mom actually videoed the entire thing because it was hilarious. Let's just say, there was a good amount of explicit language being used.

My two friends wore these devices for two days. Whenever I was low, they were drinking a juice box or eating fruit snacks as well. When I was bolusing for dinner, so were they (not actually, I took the batteries in their pumps out). I tried to make it as similar to my life as possible; however, there were still aspects of it that couldn't be captured by wearing the pump and CGM. For example they weren't getting the symptoms I was when my blood sugar was low. They ate the fruit snacks, but they didn't feel like crap the way I did.

When the weekend was over, I removed the devices they were wearing and they went home. A few hours later, one of my friends sent me this incredibly kind and thoughtful text: "Just wanted to say how proud I am of you for doing this every day. Even though I walked around with sites and pricked my finger a few times, it's not even close to what you go through on a daily basis. I'm truly amazed! I'm glad we did this because it gives me a new perspective and appreciation!"

There aren't enough words in the English language to articulate how grateful I was that my friends decided to do this. It meant the world to know that they cared. They wanted to understand what I go through and as friends, there is nothing more I could ask of them.

What Not to Say

There are so many sayings that drive Type 1 diabetics over the edge. In an effort to try and inform people about the disease, here are some sayings that annoy me (and I'm sure many others). They are not only inaccurate, but whether you realize it or not, offensive. The sad part is when people say them, they aren't trying to be rude; they just have no idea what they are talking about. I don't know how else to say it or put that nicely; it's just the way it is. So, here we go....

"Oh yeah, I know all about diabetes because my grandma has it. She just takes a shot once a day and she's totally fine."
A bunch of issues with this one, the first being that Type 1 is not like, oh let's just take a shot and I'll be fine. Not even close. So bottom line is, if you compare me to your grandma, good luck. You better start running—unless of course your grandma actually has Type 1!

"Oh, it can't be that bad because you'll just grow out of it!"

Not much needed here, expect for the fact that no, I will not "grow out of it." Unfortunately it is here to stay and I will have it for the rest of my life.

"I think I have diabetes because I ate so much sugar and junk food."

This one's pretty self-explanatory and is probably the one I despise the most. You DO NOT get Type 1 by eating sugar and junk food. It is Type 2 that has to do with lifestyle. I cannot tell you how many times I have heard this reference on TV and even in Broadway shows. Every time I hear it, it makes me want to scream!!!

"Look at this lollipop! It's diabetes on a stick!"

This is something someone said in a candy store in Vermont a couple of years ago. I think my blood pressure skyrocketed after hearing it (no, not my blood sugar, my blood *pressure*). I am not even going to tell you what's wrong here because I think you get the point about the connection, or lack thereof, between T1D and sugar.

"Oh my gosh you're a diabetic? I would have never guessed that! You don't look like a diabetic!"

No. Just no. Being a Type 1 diabetic has absolutely nothing to do with being a certain weight. Furthermore, unless you are like me and wear your pump and/or CGM visible for everyone to see, you would never know someone's a "diabetic."

This one isn't a "what not to say" I think it's just flat out hilarious....

"Type 1 diabetes brings the phrase 'human pin cushion' to a whole new level.'"

Not naming any names but one of my teachers (you know who you are) referred to me as a "human pin cushion" one day. I was dying of laughter. So hilarious and yet so true.

Celebrities

I'm sure you don't know it, but there are so many celebrities and professional athletes that have T1D. Some of them include (in no particular order):

Nick Jonas: singer/songwriter

Halle Berry: actress

Mary Tyler Moore: actress

Crystal Bowersox: singer/songwriter

Jean Smart: actress

Elliott Yamin: singer

Dorian Gregory: actor (some movies he was in include "Show Stoppers" and "Getting Played")

Bret Michaels: singer/songwriter

Anne Rice: author

Damon Dash: entrepreneur (co-founder of Roc-A-Fella Records)

Sonia Sotomayor: Associate Justice of the Supreme Court of the U.S.

Casey Johnson: actress, model, and author

Gary Hall Jr.: olympic swimmer

Victor Garber: actor

Robin Thicke - singer/songwriter

Jay Cutler - NFL player (quarterback)

Mike Echols - NFL player (cornerback)

Kendall Simmons - NFL player (guard)

Jake Byrne - NFL player (tight end)

Nicole Johnson - first Miss America to have Type 1 (she won in 1999)

These are just some of the people who are with me and so many others on this journey. I often look to them for hope. To see all of these successful athletes, actors, singers, you name it, doing so well in the world comforts me. It creates a sense of relief to know that I am not alone on this rollercoaster ride; there are others who are way more accomplished than I am who go through the same thing.

Working Out, or At Least Trying To

Still to this day, running and cardio workouts are near impossible which is frustrating. No matter what I do in advance, I still plummet a mile and a half into my run which pisses me off. I often think about the fact that it's just not fair. All of my friends can get on the treadmill or go outside and run two miles no problem, but for me it seems even the most meticulous planning is still not enough.

There was one day in particular about a year and a half ago where I lost it. I was working out with my mom; she was on the Peloton bike and I was on the treadmill. I had run a mile and a half and was aiming for at least one more when my CGM started beeping with the urgent low glucose alarm. I was so determined to run one more mile that my mom had to practically pry me off of the treadmill to get me to treat my low. My CGM said I was 50mg/dL with two arrows pointing straight down, meaning I was dropping rapidly.

I'll never forget the feeling of being pulled off of the

treadmill and lying face down on the floor. I felt so defeated. I drank a cup of juice while nearly breaking down in tears, which is a rare occurrence if there are others around me. Thinking back, that was probably the time in my life that I've felt the most helpless. I felt like such a failure. I just wanted to run one more freaking mile but apparently my mind and my body were not in agreement.

One aspect of working out with Type 1 that bothers me the most is how difficult it is to lose weight. I get frustrated because if I go for a run on the treadmill (or do any sort of physical activity for that matter), I have to drink an entire gatorade afterwards because I'm low. The fact that I then have to make up all of the calories I just burned off is infuriating, and obviously makes it that much more difficult to actually lose weight. Another reason it's so hard is anytime that I'm low, I have to eat or drink something with carbs. Often times at these moments when I need something, I'm not even hungry. So I'm basically forced to eat when I am not hungry at all and let me tell you a little secret, eating when you're not hungry doesn't exactly help you shed weight.

Lately I have been able to control my blood sugars a little better, but with way too much thought put in when all I want is to go for a damn run. Usually I take my pump off two hours prior and then while I'm running, I sip on gatorade throughout which keeps me somewhat steady. The issue is this one method does not work every time. As I've mentioned before, the inconsistency with Type 1 is the only thing that's consistent, so it definitely keeps me on my toes to say the least.

Important Figures and Music

One thing that has always been something that gets me out of bed and keeps me motivated is music. There aren't words to express how important it is to me. It has helped me through all of the ups and downs in my life. My family gets annoyed because they think all I do it listen to music. I listen in the halls at school, anytime I'm in the car, when I'm getting dressed, and while taking a shower. I generally have it maxed out when I'm driving alone, screaming the lyrics at the top of my lungs. I love music with meaningful lyrics because they inspire me to keep going when my life gets hard.

Music has picked me up when all I've wanted to do was fall down. I think part of the reason that I love it so much is because I've always envied singers. I always wanted to be able to sing without breaking glass or having my dad tell me to "shut up," but it never worked. I walk around singing my favorite artists' songs, which Caroline hates. She is constantly asking me why I sing all the time.

Since I figured out that I had just about zero chance of having a singing career, I started playing the flute in fourth grade. Throughout my childhood, I never knew why I'd be playing and listening to music all of the time but now that I think about it, it's because that's how I cope with things. I just listen to music. Music inspires me; that's exactly why I surround myself with it.

On TV as well, I always look for people who inspire me. When I first saw Jennifer Lopez on "American Idol," I automatically became a huge fan of hers. She always looked gorgeous and seemed so sweet. She also doesn't carry around the bad reputations that many other celebrities do. I Googled her music and soon enough my playlist consisted of her music, and only her music. To this day, I still blast it (in both English and Spanish) from my speaker in my room or in the shower. P.S. - her Spanish album is pretty amazing. I know all of the words to "Qué Hiciste."

As the "American Idol" seasons went by and I kept growing to love her more and more, I Googled some of her movies. Not long after, I completely fell in love with *Maid in Manhattan* and *The Wedding Planner*. Besides the fact that when Luke wanted to see the movie *Home*, the only reason I went was because she was one of the voices in it. One thing that really made me love her was that every day she would post "quotes to live by" on Facebook. I really enjoyed reading those because they gave me something to think about. They inspired me to try and make myself a better person each day.

Another hero of mine whose music has kept me going throughout my life, is Adele. I had always liked her from a young age, but one day in particular she became one of my idols.

I got a text from my mom one day saying that my dad's friend had offered him two tickets to an Adele concert. She asked me if I wanted to go. Obviously I said yes, because who doesn't want to see Adele live at Madison Square Garden? So we planned to go to her first show in New York City on a Monday night.

When the day finally came, my mom picked me up from school so I could get my homework done before we had to leave around 4:30pm. As soon as I got home from school, I got right to my homework and then when I finished, I ran upstairs to get dressed for the concert. On the drive into New York City, my mom and I figured we should probably listen to some Adele music to get ready and excited - like I wasn't excited enough already. It was kind of funny though because as I looked through my music, I realized I really only knew four or five of her songs. (Long story short, it didn't matter that I only knew "Rumor Has It," "Rolling in the Deep," "Set Fire to the Rain," "Hello," and "Send My Love to Your New Lover" going into the concert). We grabbed a quick dinner beforehand and then walked to Madison Square Garden.

I have no words to describe the concert other than absolutely incredible and life-changing. Not only does her voice sound better in person than it does on the radio (but obviously she sounds amazing there, too), but she is so personable and funny. I loved how her personality was so embedded in the concert. There were moments during it where I kid you not, my entire body was shaking because her voice is just that powerful.

I think one of the reasons that I love Jennifer Lopez and Adele so much is because they just seem like such real, down to earth people that I can relate to. They aren't afraid to be themselves. This is an extremely important characteristic in celebrities and it is rare to find nowadays.

It occurs to me now that Adele's music in particular has a profound effect on me. Some say her music is depressing, but it is exactly what I need to listen to when I'm having a bad day because it reminds me that I'm not the only one who has to go through tough times. Music serves as a source of comfort for me. It keeps me grounded and looking in the right direction.

In the Public Eye

Facing the real world with people who don't have any idea what T1D is like is difficult. I completely understand what is must be like to see someone like me in public because I don't try to hide anything. When I walk around in shorts during the summer with my insulin pump on one leg, and CGM on the other, it looks really weird. I'm sure to others, I look like a spy working for the FBI. My hygienist in the dentist's office asked me one time if I was a bionic woman. That was a little strange considering she was a grown adult. Not going to lie, it was pretty funny though.

Kids, adults, teenagers, they all wonder and they all stare. It's part of our nature as human beings. If we don't see something recognizable, we look intensely to try and figure out what it is; I am completely understanding of that. Yes, it's a little uncomfortable walking around with everyone staring at me, but I want to show people that it's good to be different. There are going to be people with disabilities and diseases in the world, and our ridiculously judgmental society needs to learn to accept that.

I will never forget the time where I was on the bus ride home of my first day in high school. I went to school in a nice shirt and shorts with my insulin pump on one leg, CGM on the other. There were seniors on the bus who were staring at me. So I politely addressed them by asking if they had any questions (thinking back that was oddly bold of me as a little freshman on the first day of school but whatever). They replied by saying, "What the hell's on your legs?" As this was not a very nice comment, I kept my cool and explained to them what the "gadgets" were, and what their functions are. Afterwards, they loosened up a bit by saying, "Oh, that's cool." It made me happy that I was able to advocate to older kids about my disease and raise awareness for people with T1D.

Although I wasn't exactly laughing about it at the time, today I find the whole situation hilarious. I am thrilled that I feel comfortable enough in my own skin to advocate for myself and everyone living with this disease.

One of the main reasons I decided to write this book is because I want to educate people as to what Type 1 is and what it entails. I also want people to know that a key part of being happy is being comfortable in your own skin. Everyone goes through shit in life. Sometimes it's visible and sometimes it's not. But you need to be so confident that you don't give a crap what people think of you. If people want to be jerks and not accept you for who you are, let them. That's their loss, not yours.

Not Every Day Can Be Sunny

As I mentioned before, there are definitely some days that just flat out suck. There are two in particular that stand out in my mind; the first one took place when I was at my cousins' house in Lake George. Every other year we go up to Lake George for Thanksgiving weekend. It's really nice because all of my cousins, aunts, and uncles are there, so it's great being able to spend time with them considering we don't see them much during the year.

One year after eating our delicious Thanksgiving dinner, my cousins and I decided that we wanted to go Black Friday shopping. We left around 11pm and we drove half an hour to the outlets. My blood sugar had been a little high prior to leaving, but I assumed that was just because of an error when I was estimating the number of carbs on my plate.

In the car on the way to the outlets, I remember having my phone open to the Dexcom app where I can see my blood sugars. I watched it climb for twenty minutes. I had started around 210mg/dL and by that point I was 330mg/dL and headed up really fast, as denoted by the two up arrows on my phone. My head started pounding, but I knew I had to rally so I gave myself an absurd amount of insulin as a correction and carried on with my cousins. I figured my blood sugar should start to come down about an hour later, so I told myself I would wait until then.

Soon enough that hour came to a close. I opened the app on my phone and was in complete shock at what I saw. My CGM now said "HIGH" with two arrows pointed up. At this point my head was pounding and I felt horrible, but I couldn't tell my cousins I needed to go back home; they had waited all day for this and we had just gotten there. I recall being so frustrated that the initial correction I gave myself didn't work. I gave myself more insulin and tried to carry on. This is when I started to get a little confused. Sometimes my guessing skills aren't phenomenal, but I was certain that I was not this off. There was no way. If anything, I had given myself too much insulin. As these thoughts were running through my head on repeat, I realized that it must be my infusion site. I told my cousins I was going to the bathroom. There, I took the cartridge of insulin out of my pump and took out eight units with one of the syringes I always carry for this exact reason. I gave myself a shot and tried to convince myself that soon enough I'd be home in bed, the only place I wanted to be at the time.

While we were shopping, I was trying my best to suck it up and pretend everything was fine while on the inside I was physically and mentally exhausted.

My blood sugar started to drop two hours after my shot,

and we arrived back home around 3am. When we got back to the house, even though all I wanted was to sleep for a year, I had to do a new site since mine had clearly failed. I did that as quickly but accurately as I could, and went right to bed, hoping I would sleep off this horrible feeling.

I woke up the next morning feeling so much better, and I explained to my cousins the situation that had occurred the night prior. They felt terrible and told me I should've told them, but I didn't want to ruin their night just because of my disease. It wasn't fair to them. But in hindsight, I probably should have told them what was going on just to make them aware, considering that with the extremely high blood sugars I was experiencing, I was not far away from being hospitalized. I knew I should have told them, but I didn't want my medical problems to be a burden for them. This is my shit that I have to deal with, and the last thing I wanted to do was share the added stress with them.

The second day that stands out in my mind is one from my family vacation in Nantucket one year. My family plus my best friend, Colleen, and my aunt's family were out to dinner in a restaurant called The Brotherhood. Colleen is the adopted child in my house, so often times when I'm referring to "my family," Colleen is included in that reference. Everything was great; we were having a nice normal meal. When we were getting ready to pay, I noticed my blood sugar was 75mg/dL and heading down quickly. I thought that was odd considering I'd just eaten dinner. My dad ordered me a Coke and said to drink that until we got to The Juice Bar, objectively the best ice cream shop on the island.

I drank the Coke immediately, but fifteen minutes later when we were ready to leave, I felt significantly worse than I had initially. I knew it was a short walk, so I figured I would walk over and by then the Coke would start working. When I stood up to walk, I felt light-headed, another symptom of being low. I tried to not make it a big deal, but when I got to the stairs it hit me. I was a whole lot lower than 75mg/dL. My vision started to go, and by the time I made it down the stairs by grasping the hand rail and taking it one step at a time, I had almost lost my vision completely. The things I could see were extremely blurry, and I felt like I was going to pass out. My mom and aunt were holding me up and helping me walk until we got to the nearest bench.

My aunt stayed with me while my mom sprinted to the closest store to buy me yet another Coke. She uncapped it and said to drink as much as I could. I was so nauseous that I couldn't eat or drink anything but I didn't exactly have a choice. I took one tiny sip at a time, nearly vomiting after each one. Eventually, I finished the whole soda and started to feel better twenty-five minutes later.

The part I remember most about that day was the feeling. Besides being scared out of my mind, it was the worst I've ever felt; the lack of vision, shaking, sweating. I genuinely thought I was going to die. The part that was freaking me out was that my mom was panicking, because she is one of the most laid-back people in the world. When my mom's freaking out, you know you have a reason to be worried.

Overall I consider myself a fairly positive person because I believe that your attitude dictates your happiness in life.

Reflecting on these days now makes me realize that everyone goes through tough days no matter how positive your attitude is. But the days where you feel like your life is ending are the ones where you have to be the strongest. I've learned that when I'm angry or annoyed at T1D, I need to go somewhere alone, cry it out, and then carry on with my life. It's acceptable to be upset, but letting the frustration take you over is not. You have to let it be your motivation to come out stronger tomorrow.

My Average Day

My average day is definitely nothing less than a nightmare. But you know what? This is what God gave to me so I am going to take what I have and run with it. My motto is: never let anything get the best of you. You were put where you are now for a reason, so the best thing you can do is deal with it, be brave, and have a positive attitude.

To give you a better idea of my day to day routine and to help you understand what I (and many others) deal with, here is what my average day looked like on a weekday and weekend in high school. I decided that giving you a look into my high school life would be easier because my life in college varies from day to day and is much more chaotic.

Weekday:

First things first, my alarm is set for 7am. I am an early riser and feel that if I wake up late, I am missing part of the day so needless to say, I wake up early. On Mondays, Wednesdays, and Fridays I get up around 5:45am and workout before school. On Tuesdays and Thursdays, I am usually up at about 6:30 or 6:45am. I'm sure you think I'm insane right now, but I forgot to mention one minor detail that is going to do nothing but confuse you more. I may have forgotten to say that I go to bed very early for someone my age. On weekdays I'm sleeping between 9 and 9:30pm the latest. I just feel like if I go to bed early, then I can wake up early and see the sun rise. ("The sky's awake, so I'm awake, so we have to play!" Where are my "Frozen" fans? Shoot, I really need to "let it go." Sorry, it was the perfect opportunity!). Plus, I work better in the morning. For the six on and off years I've been writing this book, I would wake up super early and just write. I would write for an hour or two before my alarm went off, and I got so much done. It made me feel like I accomplished so much at 7am!

Anyway, back to my day. After my alarm goes off, I get out of bed, brush my teeth, and take my thyroid pill. Afterwards I get dressed, brush my hair, and all that fun stuff. Then, I go downstairs and check my blood sugar for the second time of the day (this is only 7am!). The first time is right when I wake up and look at my phone. Sometimes I eat breakfast, but not usually. I'm one of those people who feel sick when they eat breakfast. I leave my house at 7:45am, get to school around 7:55am, and get right to class. I always wear my apple watch because if my blood sugar is high or low, it can alert me since it is connected to my CGM. I know, pretty freaking cool. I constantly check my blood sugar throughout the day; usually once or twice per period (each one is forty minutes). When I get to lunch I test my blood sugar, then give myself insulin for my meal. After the rest of my afternoon classes, I head straight to the barn to ride Gideon.

When I get to the barn I change my clothes, groom and brush Gideon, and tack him up. I have to check my blood sugar to make sure I won't go low various times while I'm at the barn. I check when I arrive, right before I get on, after I ride, and before I go home. Typically, I have Swedish fish or Welch's fruit snacks prior to getting on, but I always have to keep an eye on it to make sure I don't go low while on horseback. I normally ride Gideon for around forty-five minutes, then untack him and brush him off (or bathe him if it's a hot day). I go home around 5:45pm, do my homework, take a shower, and eat dinner. By then it's around 8:15pm, so I make my chamomile tea and go watch Netflix in bed. The weekdays are not as hard since I have a routine, but I'm willing to bet it's a lot more thought and attention to health than most others' average day.

Weekend:

Usually on the weekends, I wake up around 6:30am and go downstairs to catch up on my favorite shows. It's usually either "Law and Order: SVU," (my absolute favorite!! Liv is the best!) "Grey's Anatomy," or "Riverdale." By 8:30am, I am upstairs getting dressed for a day at the barn. I make my lunch, and then I'm on my way by 9am (unless it's Sunday, then I go to church first).

When I get there, I immediately get to work. On the weekends, I usually ride quite a few horses; most of the time with no *break to eat lunch. I enjoy it though, so it's completely worth it. Before I begin working with every horse, I check my blood sugar and treat it accordingly. It is incredible that my parents have the faith to leave me at the barn all day knowing my life is literally in my own hands.*

After all of my riding for the day is done, I go home, take a shower and just relax for the rest of the day. Sometimes I run errands with my mom, help her cook dinner, or whatever else my family is doing on that particular day (during the winter it's watch football for the entire afternoon).

Although Type 1 is second nature to me, I still have to think about it and make decisions all day every day no matter what I'm doing. As I've said over and over again, the tough part is that there is no consistency. Every single day is totally different from the one prior. T1D is an unpredictable disease that never stays the same, which makes it so damn difficult.

After writing down what my average day entails, I have realized what an effect this disease has on me. Because I don't really remember living without it, I don't pay attention to how much extra worry and stress is added to my life. Even though it doesn't seem fair, I constantly have to remind myself that there is a reason I'm in the situation I'm in right now. God has instilled His trust in me to manage this and fight for my life. He is the reason that I have the strength to do this every single day.

Marshall and Sterling Finals

As you already know, I'm a big equestrian. If you didn't know that, then you have not been paying attention (just kidding!). A little background on Gideon…I got him when he was very young and I have been training him ever since. Before Gideon, I had a horse named Vancouver. I owe a ton to him. He taught me how to ride.

In 2013, I qualified for Marshall and Sterling National Finals with Vancouver. These finals take the top forty riders in each division from around the country, and they compete. In 2013, I qualified for these finals and out of the top forty riders in my 2'6" jumping division (for you riders it was the Children's Medal), I placed fourth. It was incredible, to say the least. I cannot thank Vancouver enough for everything he has done for me. Unfortunately, we ended up donating him to an all-girls boarding school in Massachusetts due to a reoccurring injury making it difficult to sell him.

The following year, I had just gotten Gideon and was

training him, so we did not show enough to qualify in 2014. However, in 2015 I qualified and took Gideon to Marshall and Sterling Finals. This time, I was competing in the 3' jumping division (once again, for you horse people it was the Children's Hunter Classic). I ended up placing seventh in one class and eighth in the other. It was the most amazing feeling knowing that I trained him to be the horse he was in order to place seventh out of the top horses and riders in my division. It was also such a huge step for both him and me because when I got him, he didn't have much experience at all because he was so young. I was so proud of him that day. I must have given him five apples (and a lot of Welch's fruit snacks!).

Riding has not only given me a sport where I feel like I am not being limited by Type 1, but it has taught me so many important life lessons. My experience training Gideon has taught me that hard work really does pay off. Although we had our obstacles along the way, the patience I gained from training him assisted in developing me as a person. There is no doubt in my mind that training him was one of the most difficult tasks I've ever even attempted. There were some days where I would try to teach him something and he would just get it, but there were plenty of other days where it took hours for him to understand what I was trying to tell him. It's not exactly like I could use words to tell him what I wanted! I also learned that I can do anything I set my mind to, no matter how hard it may seem at times. Dreams can be a reality. The deciding factor on whether they are or not, is simply how hard you're willing to work.

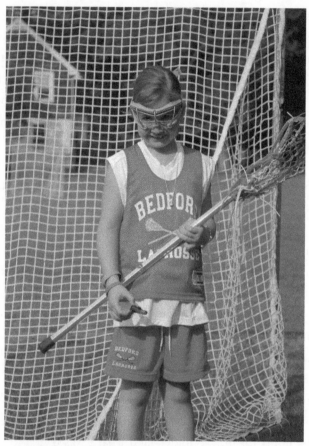

My first time playing lacrosse at just seven years old!

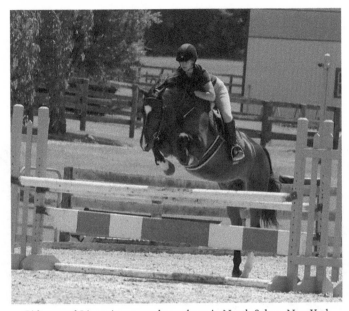

Gideon and I jumping at our home barn in North Salem, New York
one day after school.

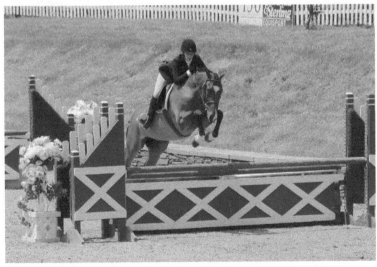

Taking advantage of a nice day of showing at HITS Saugerties
one summer.

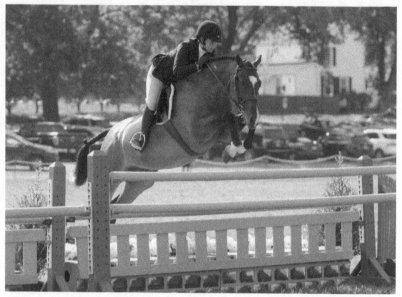

Gideon and me showing, at Fairfield County Hunt Club in
Westport, Connecticut.
Picture Credits: Amanda Ward

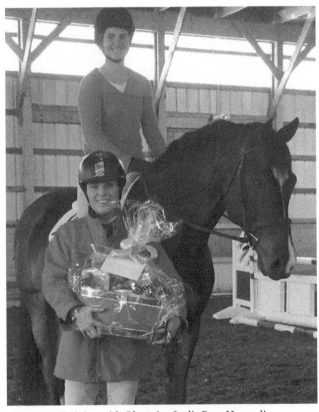

Training with Olympian Leslie Burr Howard!

Part IV

"The one who falls and gets up is so much stronger than
the one who never fell."

ANONYMOUS

Dean's House

My dad works closely with some very impressive people; one being Dean Kamen. Dean is an entrepreneur and inventor who designed and engineered his own insulin pump. In 2001, he invented the Segway, which is basically a hoverboard with a stick in the front. Among many other things, he also invented the iBOT wheelchair; a wheelchair that can climb stairs.

One day, my dad came home from work and said to me, "I know a really cool guy and he wants to meet you. Would you come up to his house with me one night and stay over? His name's Dean Kamen." I immediately Googled him, and all of his inventions popped up. He seemed like an amazing guy. Shortly thereafter, I agreed to go.

I was in eighth grade at the time, so luckily it wasn't a big deal to miss a day of school. So one Friday I took the day off and my dad and I drove up to Dean's house. When we got there, we went up to the door where a very nice lady greeted us. She told us Dean would be with us in a moment. Right inside the entrance of his house, there was a huge steam engine. And by huge, I'm talking HUGE. When Dean came out, he shook my hand and said, "It's a pleasure to meet you. Let me show you around my house." First, he started telling me about this massive steam engine. He said that it was the first real steam engine to be used in America and when he got it, it was not in very good shape. So he decided to take it apart, restore it, and then put it back together.

After showing me around his beautiful, yet eclectic house with his inventions and awards everywhere, it was time for dinner. Dean's chef cooked us a delicious five-course meal which I ate way too much of. I swear I was full for the next three days! After dinner, he showed me his helicopter in his garage. Yes, you read that correctly. In designing the house, he put in an extra garage big enough to fit a helicopter. Because he actually built this helicopter himself, he flew to work in it every day. When he showed it to me, he said, "This is what we're flying to work in tomorrow." I didn't know how to respond because I was just in awe, still trying to get over the fact that he had a helicopter in his house.

The next morning I woke up, got dressed, and went downstairs. While my dad and I were eating breakfast, I asked him where Dean was. He said that he was getting ready. All of a sudden while we were eating, out walked Dean from the kitchen cabinet. "What the heck are you doing walking out of the kitchen cabinet?" my dad asked. Dean then went on to explain that when he was little, he wanted to have a house similar to one you could read about or watch in cartoons;

like the ones where you could pull a book out of the bookshelf and there's a secret room. So when he was creating the plans for his house, he designed it with a book that you pull out of the shelf in his library, and up comes a secret room. This theory also explained why he walked out of the kitchen cabinet that morning.

After eating breakfast and witnessing Dean walking out of his cabinet, which had already been an eventful day by 8am, it was time to go to work. My dad, Dean, and I went into his "garage" where his helicopter was. I got in, and he gave me headphones to put on (you know, the ones that pilots of helicopters wear). We took off in the helicopter and he flew us to one of his office buildings. Once we got there, which, by the way, took five minutes compared to a twenty-minute drive in a car, we were hovering over the roof. "What are we doing?" my dad asked.

"Landing," Dean replied. With that, we landed on the roof of Dean Kamen's office building in his helicopter that he built himself.

We went into the office building where I met his assistant Julie, and then we went into a meeting. As I mentioned before, Dean invented his own insulin pump for people with Type 1, so he was showing my dad and me the model that had just come in. It was fascinating to sit there with all of these talented engineers and listen to the future technology that was eventually going to come out to help people with Type 1. After the meeting was over, my dad and I said goodbye. Then unfortunately, it was time to drive home.

When I got home, I told my mom and siblings about all of the crazy things that had happened while at Dean's house. Looking back now, not only was it an unforgettable experience, but it is so admirable that Dean is working on a massive project to help people with a disease that he has no connection to. I owe a huge thank you to Dean Kamen for showing me everything he did, and for trying to make life in the T1D world so much easier. It goes to show you that there are always good people in the world who are eager to help; all you need to do is ask.

Behind the Scenes

There are some things that make living with Type 1 really tricky. It's the things that you normally would never think twice about. For example, going through airport security. Do not get me started on airport security. Well, now that I mentioned it, I'll tell you why airport security is every Type 1 diabetic's worst nightmare.

So you know how when you're traveling, you put your carry-on bags through that machine, then you walk through the big metal detector and you're on your way in five minutes maximum (not including the line of course)? Well it is not that simple for people with Type 1. First of all, my bag always beeps because it has needles, juice, and all kinds of stuff that you're normally not allowed to bring on a plane. Then I beep when I walk through the metal detector because of my pump, which creates a whole separate mess. The technician then asks me to "step aside" to come talk to them. This is generally how it goes down….

Security technician: "Is there anything in this bag that could harm me?"

Me: "Yes. There are needles in there because I am a Type 1 diabetic." *Gives the security technician the doctor's note saying that I am allowed to bring anything necessary on the plane*

Security technician: *Searches my bag and pulls my juice out* "You're not allowed to bring this on the plane. You have to buy something once you get through security."

Me: "I'm not sure what part you're not understanding. I must bring this in case of an emergency. If you really have a problem, then call my doctor. His number is on the note."

Security technician: "Then we will have to wipe down each one of these fifteen juice boxes to make sure there's no gun powder or anything in them."

Me: "Go for it."

Security technician: *After wiping down fifteen juice boxes one by one* "Now you have to come for a pat down."

Then they bring me off to the side to do this very invasive and uncomfortable pat down. Not only is it invasive, but it is time-consuming. Bottom line is, the security in an airport that normally takes less than five minutes becomes a twenty-five minute ordeal for me. I understand that they are doing their job and they just want to make sure I'm not going to harm anyone on the plane, but it is very frustrating, especially because they generally aren't nice about it. Maybe it's the lack of education that makes it difficult.

Hopefully this situation will improve and the security technicians will show more compassion and knowledge as they start seeing more and more people with Type 1. The number of people with the disease is rising rapidly, so in theory you would expect the number of people traveling with Type 1 to increase, too, but only time will tell.

Helping the New Victims

Ever since I was diagnosed and my dad became extremely involved in the care and management of T1D, anyone who was diagnosed in our family or friends' families was sent to us. We always try to help as best as we can because we have been through it, and know how difficult the beginning is.

The day before our spring break in March of 2016 when I was in ninth grade, my English teacher, Mrs. Whitbourne, was absent from school. My friend, who was in my English class, came in and told me that Mrs. Whitbourne's son, who was seven years old, had just been diagnosed with Type 1 diabetes. She knew because her mom was also an English teacher at our school and was friendly with Mrs. Whitbourne. Once I heard that her son Brendan was diagnosed, I immediately texted my mom and asked her to reach out to the Whitbourne family to see if they needed any help or support. My parents offered for Mrs. Whitbourne and her family to come over to our house, so we could show them the ropes and help them understand what the future had in store.

The day they were supposed to come over, I rode Gideon in the morning, took a shower and helped my mom clean the house before they came. When they arrived, we talked to them to see how Brendan was handling the finger pricks, shots, and all of that kind of stuff. Mrs. Whitbourne and her husband told us that he was such a trooper and was doing a great job. That was awesome for me to hear because when I was diagnosed just a year younger than he was, I was a complete disaster. The Whitbournes stayed for a few hours while we explained the basics. I also showed Brendan my pump and I told him that when he was able to get it, his life would be so much easier.

One of the few things I love about T1D is that it gives me the opportunity to help all of those who are newly diagnosed. Shortly after my diagnosis, my parents and I met with a family who had a daughter my age with Type 1. It was so comforting to have someone there to tell us that it wasn't necessarily going to be okay, but that it's manageable for the most part. I think this experience was what made me want to help all of the newly diagnosed. I thoroughly enjoy educating people and trying to calm their nerves, which I think is part of the reason that I am studying biology to be a pediatric endocrinologist.

I just recently thought about the reciprocation aspect of this act. If I need people in my life to support me through the times when Type 1 is kicking my ass, then I need to be there to help others when they are going through the same situation. I feel like support is more meaningful when you have someone who has already been through what you're going through, telling you that it does get better. I like to think that it provides at least some sense of encouragement when everything else in your life seems like hell.

Robin and Rome

One night at a restaurant called Mama Rosa, near my house, my dad got an email from the CEO of an organization called Stem for Life. If you've never heard of the Stem for Life Foundation, it is basically an organization that was established to educate the general population about stem cell research and just gain more support for the cause. The CEO asked if I would be on a panel with my dad in Rome to speak about Type 1 diabetes. They host this event every other year and it is held in Vatican City. As my dad gathered more information, he found out that he, my mom, Caroline, and I would all speak on the panel in front of a few hundred people to discuss what it was like living with T1D. Our moderator would be ABC's anchor for *Good Morning America*, Robin Roberts. The Pope was also expected to possibly make an appearance.

I contemplated the idea because I used to be petrified of public speaking. But the more I thought about it, I realized that it would be the opportunity of a lifetime. Shortly thereafter, my family and I booked our trip. We were going to be in Italy from a Tuesday to Sunday, as our panel was supposed to be Thursday and the conference ran from Thursday to Saturday. Our trip was scheduled for the last week of April.

During the end of March, we set up a time to meet with Robin Roberts prior to the event so we could get a better idea of what kinds of questions she was going to ask us. We scheduled a date to go into New York City to the *Good Morning America* set and watch the morning show. It was amazing to see everything that goes into making a TV show. As we watched from behind the scenes, Robin's assistant, Reni, came over and explained to us everything that was going on.

Days before meeting Robin, I had Googled her to get some background information, so I wasn't totally in the dark. I quickly found out that just years prior, she suffered from breast cancer, which then led to Myelodysplastic Syndrome (MDS), requiring a bone marrow transplant. After reading this information, I was so anxious to meet this incredibly strong woman.

We took the train into New York City the morning of the show, and then walked to the building they were filming in. While we were standing next to the set, Robin came over and introduced herself. Speaking to her was very inspiring. I remember wondering how one could go through such tragedy in their life and end up as amazing and positive as Robin. We talked for a few minutes and then she said something. Something that stuck with me. Robin said that when she had cancer and decided to keep it private rather than releasing it to the public, her mom said something to her that changed her mind. Her mom told her, "Make your mess, your message." She then followed it up by saying that she was very proud of me. She told me that I was making a difference and touching people's lives. This has been all I have been aiming to do throughout my years with this disease and for freaking Robin Roberts to tell me I was accomplishing my dream was absolutely incredible!

In retrospect, meeting Robin Roberts was eye-opening. After hearing her story and now thinking back on it years later, I think the most important lesson I learned that day is that there is always someone in this world who is going through something worse than you. I also realize that I am contradicting previous statements I've made. I have said that Type 1 sucks and that it affects every single aspect of my life, which it does. But I also understand how lucky I am. I'm lucky that I live where I do. I'm lucky that I have running water and food on the table. So yes, T1D is a brutal disease and it knocks me down more days than I can count, but I am lucky that for the time being, this is the only thing I have to worry about. It's made me think deeply every time I complain about something small.

The Trip of a Lifetime

The day it all began, I got picked up from school at 12:00pm on a Tuesday and we were off to the airport. Our flight was scheduled to depart from Newark Airport at 5:00pm, so we started boarding at 4:15pm.

Eight hours of flying later, we went to our hotel in Rome. At age fifteen I wrote, *Wow were the rooms there beautiful! We had three connecting rooms, one for my parents, one for Caroline, Luke, and me, and one for Mimi. They were gorgeous with incredible views from the balcony overlooking the city.*

We got settled into our room and then went to have lunch upstairs in the hotel. We ran into Gary Hall Jr., an Olympic swimmer with T1D, so we wound up having lunch with him. Gary is pretty amazing. He's won ten Olympic medals, five of which are gold. Oh and he's done all of that with Type 1. Needless to say, having the privilege of eating lunch with Gary was a fantastic start to our trip.

After lunch, we went on an adventure to explore the city

for a bit. It was incredible to look at all of the gorgeous architecture and think about the fact that it was hand-carved.

By the time we got back to the hotel, we were all pretty shot from a long day of traveling, so we took a short nap and went out to dinner. And if you haven't been to Italy...yes, the food is AMAZING! We ate at this little restaurant near the Spanish Steps before crashing for twelve hours that night. I had the best linguine carbonara of my life. I get hungry just thinking about it.

On Thursday morning we got a quick breakfast and then were back in the heart of Rome doing some more sightseeing. We visited the Colosseum and the Parliament, both of which were breath-taking. All of the architecture in Rome is beautiful and it has so much history behind it, too. We had our interview with Robin later that day, so we couldn't stay out for too long before heading back to the hotel to get ready.

Once we got back, I got dressed, straightened my hair, and put some makeup on. When we were all dressed and ready to go, we headed down to the lobby to get our shuttle into Vatican City where the conference was being held.

When our shuttle arrived at the Vatican, we were escorted into a gorgeous room with stadium seating and what I would call an "interview table." It's pretty much a long table with a bunch of chairs, microphones, and computers in front of each seat. We watched some of the presenters before us. This included people who were all older than me (by at least twenty-five years). We also watched some of the most intelligent scientists, doctors, and researchers in the world. Now that is what you call intimidating.

My family and I had a small private interview with the medical correspondent from CBS, Dr. Max Gomez, before our interview with Robin. While we were getting ready for our interview with Dr. Gomez, they put mics on us (which made me feel very professional and like a movie star...I was loving it!). They also had three big scary TV cameras. We went into the room with Max and all of the camera men. He started asking us questions one by one. His questions were along the lines of "What is it like living with Type 1 diabetes?" or "I'm sure you know the complications the disease can cause, does this scare you?" For those of you who don't know, if you don't take care of yourself, the complications of T1D are horrific. They include but are not limited to: blindness, nerve damage, kidney damage, heart disease, and amputated limbs; the list goes on from there. I answered Dr. Gomez's question by saying that no, I am not scared. I don't really think about that too much because I like to live in the moment and just appreciate the present day. I don't need to be thinking about the (hopefully) far away future.

After our interview with Dr. Gomez, we had a little bit of time to sit in the audience and watch before we had to go the dressing room to get ready. We listened to all of the speakers from around the world talk about new ways for management and potential cures for rare diseases. As I was sitting there, fascinated with what was being said, I remembered that I had left my extensive notes in our hotel room, which, prior to that moment, had been the only thing putting my mind at ease. You can imagine how quickly my stomach was churning after remembering that minor detail.

When it was time for our panel, Robin went out first to introduce our family. My family and I were then walked out by a staff member and we all sat in our assigned seats. I was completely quivering, petrified of what was to come. At the right hand corner of the computer screen in front of us, it had the time remaining counting down to zero. It started at twenty-five minutes. I remember thinking that those twenty-five minutes were going to be the longest ones of my life.

Before Robin started with her questions, she cracked a few jokes to wake up the audience. We were the last panel of the day so at that point, half of them were looking lethargic. Once the audience members were somewhat awake, she started with her questions. I had the first one. I was now shaking and sweating. Legitimately. I forgot exactly what the first question was, but I remember answering it and then taking a breath because I didn't sound like a complete idiot (or so I thought anyway). Then she asked my parents a few questions about how they were feeling when I was diagnosed. Caroline also had a few questions about if she was scared to potentially get T1D (at the time it was potentially…). After she answered, Robin asked me the following question: "What would you tell researchers and companies working on this disease?"

I responded by saying, "Hurry up!" And then I explained

that I would like a cure, but I am not sure that is possible in my lifetime. I also made sure to tell the audience that I really appreciated all of the hard work these amazing people were doing. Their work really has paid off! Now I have so many new gadgets and technologies, which have been truly life-changing.

Here's when the entire situation shifts from being horrifying to comical. One of the next questions—I'm not going to lie—was a little confusing. Luckily for me, Robin asked my dad his thoughts first (phew!). After listening to his answer, I kind of piggy-backed off of what he said. Then, Robin asked my mom her thoughts. These were her words exactly, "Um, uh, hm, I'm so sorry, there was a lot said between the question and now, would you mind repeating it?" Now that had the audience crying in laughter. I remember not being able to look at Caroline because she was laughing so hard and every time I looked at her, I would start laughing again. The old saying stands true: "Everything is funnier when you're not allowed to laugh."

Another highlight was when I was the one looking like a moron. Robin decided to throw in a curveball that, to be clear, was not one of the questions she initially told me she was going to ask. But in all fairness, it wasn't exactly a tricky one. I'm just an idiot. I forget how on Earth this came up, but we got to the point where Robin asked me what I like to do on the beach (I know completely unrelated, but it did happen). In this moment, a few different things popped into my head. The first being: why in the world was Robin asking me this question? Before I could stop my mouth from moving, I said, "Play…really…fun…games," with awkward pauses in between every word, instead of "tan or swim" like any normal person. But don't judge me yet; I promise there is a backstory! My family is pretty fidgety. We are not good at just sitting still for extended periods of time (especially my dad); we always have to be doing something active. Generally our game of choice is Kadima (the game with the two wooden rackets and the little plastic ball that you hit back and forth to each other. Don't deny it. You know exactly what I'm talking about). I was originally going to say "Play Kadima," but I figured all of those smart scientists and doctors may not know what that is. The outcome of this scenario was me sounding like a complete and utter moron by saying that on the beach, "We play really fun games." Yes, I know, it's really damn embarrassing.

After I was finished embarrassing myself in our interview, we went out to dinner with our friends, Dana and Phil, who were also in Italy for the conference. By the time we finished dinner, it was 10:00pm and we were tired from a long and mentally exhausting day. Well, I was exhausted anyway because that's past my bedtime on a good day!

The Friday that we were in Italy is definitely in the top three best days of my life. When we arrived in Vatican City for day two, there were still panels going on from the morning session, so we watched a few of those. We were told there was a special guest expected to make an appearance at 11:00am. Once 10:30am rolled around, we went into a huge auditorium-like room, with hundreds of chairs and a raised stage in the front. There were two sections to the seating arrangements; one right below the stage and one behind a barrier. We located our family's name in the second row right below the stage, so we were in the very front. Once we got settled, the special guests proceeded to the stage. The first, was Joe Biden. He came out and gave a moving speech about the need for research and financial support for rare diseases like the ones being highlighted at the conference.

Not long after Biden's speech, a noticeable hush came over the audience and there was a lot of whispering. The second special guest was ready to come out after being introduced by Joe Biden. It was none other than Pope Francis! The Holy Father was escorted out and suddenly there was security surrounding the stage. When it was time for the Pope's speech, we all put headphones on and there was a voice translating it from Italian to English. His speech was also incredibly inspiring. He talked mostly about everything that is occurring in the real world versus what should be occurring to help these diseases and people all around the globe.

After his thirty-minute speech, Pope Francis came over, shook hands with everyone in front of the barrier, and gave us all a pair of blessed Rosary beads. He also awarded me the Pontifical Hero Award! It was such an amazing moment. I honestly don't even know how to describe it. It felt like God himself had come down from Heaven. The way he looked me in the eye was just so surreal. My grandma, being such a devout Catholic, started crying which is completely understandable because WE HAD JUST MET THE POPE!!!!

After Pope Francis left, we had some time to speak with Joe Biden. What a nice man. My dad was telling him about my story with T1D and he was so supportive. I remember he asked me how old I was. I almost forgot because I was so in awe of everything I had just experienced. He said, "How old are you angel?" I almost said twelve! I don't even know why, probably because it was the first number that came to my mind. When it was time to go, he said, "It was so nice to meet you young lady. And remember, no real men 'til you're thirty!" I thought that was pretty funny.

We then spoke to Katie Couric, a Global News Anchor, because she was going to moderate a panel with my dad the next morning. She, too, was so supportive of the conference's mission to help people with rare, chronic diseases.

My dad's panel about philanthropy wasn't scheduled until Saturday, so we went back to the conference to watch him that morning. We got to spend a lot of time with Katie Couric, since she was my dad's moderator. Later that day, we went back to the hotel and explored Rome a bit more before returning to Vatican City for a private tour of Saint Peter's Basilica. It was not open to the public, only our conference, so we were the only people in the building. It was absolutely stunning. All of the architecture and attention to detail on both the inside and outside was unbelievable. The fact that everything was hand-carved and painted amazed me yet again. After the tour, we went back to the hotel for dinner and a movie with my grandma. My parents went to the Sistine Chapel where the Edge from the band U2 was performing (kids weren't allowed to go since there would be alcohol). My mom and dad said it was awesome. And besides, that was history made right there because the Edge was named the first pop artist to perform in the Sistine Chapel.

Unfortunately, when we woke up the next morning it was time to go home. It was a short, but sweet trip. Just five days, and they flew by with all of our once-in-a-lifetime experiences.

I understand now just how unique this opportunity truly was. Most people never even get to see the Pope in their life-time and here I was at fifteen years old being presented an award by Him. Trying to describe what I was feeling even now is proving to be impossible. My experience in Italy changed my life in that it strengthened my faith immensely. I think this was the first time I fully understood the impor-tance and power of religion in my life. I've said it before and I'll say it again: my faith in God is the reason that I wake up every day ready to fight with every ounce of my body. He has taught me that I was put in this situation for a reason, so giving up is never an option. To be able to have something that plays such a key role in my life strengthened in ways I never knew possible, completely opened my eyes.

I am eternally grateful to the Stem for Life Foundation and everyone involved for giving me this tremendous oppor-tunity. It still all feels like one huge dream.

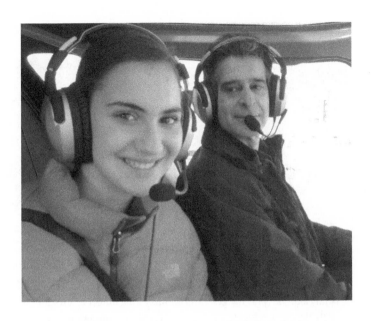

Dean Kamen and I in his garage — for his helicopter, that is!

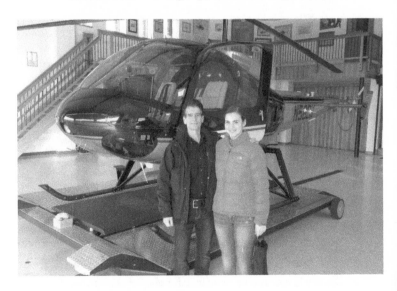

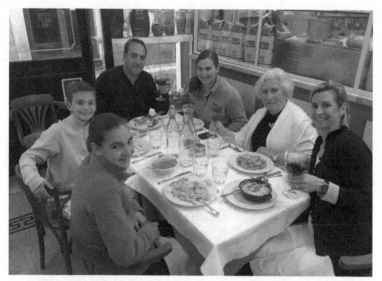

My family and me (plus my grandma, Mimi) eating dinner at a restaurant in Italy the night before our interview. This picture was taken before I started getting nauseous because I was so nervous for the interview!

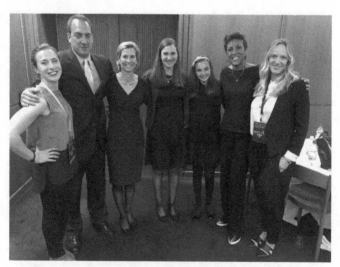

Chilling in the dressing room in Italy right after our interview. Man was I relieved! From left to right: Reni (Robin's assistant), my dad, my mom, me, Caroline, Robin, and Amber (Robin's partner).

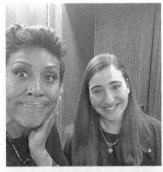

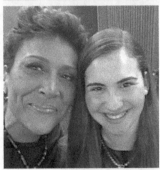

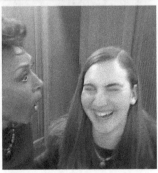

Robin and I having some post-interview fun and
taking some nice selfies.
P.S. The funny faces were all Robin's idea!

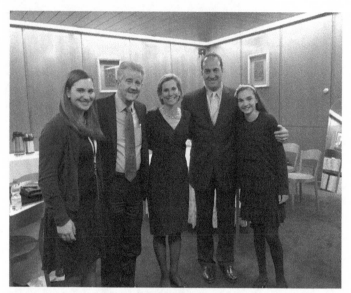

Here we are with CBS Medical Correspondent Max Gomez!

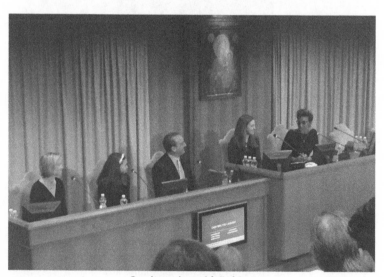

Our interview with Robin.

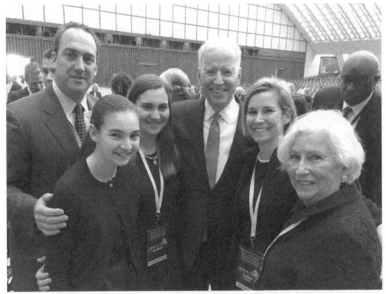

My family and I posing with former Vice President Joe Biden.

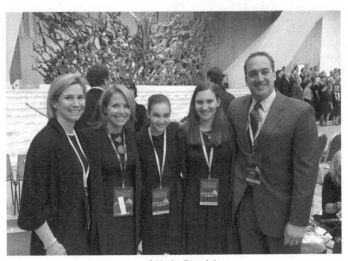

And Katie Couric!

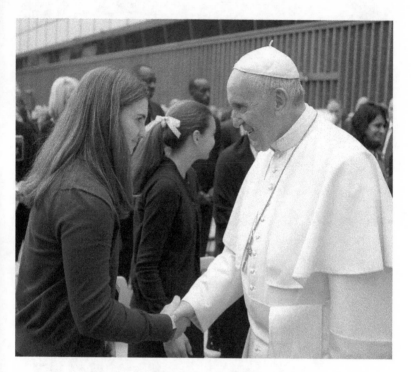

The most unforgettable of them all…
Pope Francis!

Part V

"The greater your storm the brighter the rainbow."

ANONYMOUS

Children's Congress, Take 2

As I've mentioned many times before, my dad works closely with JDRF, which is the same organization that runs the Children's Congress event I went to back in 2009. Because I already went to lobby Congress for more funding in the past, I was not allowed to go back again as a delegate. But one day, I got an email from the head of Children's Congress asking me to come speak in the opening event of the weekend; they wanted me to talk about riding competitively with T1D. I agreed to come to Washington D.C., figuring it would be a great opportunity to inspire others battling Type 1.

The event was in late July, so I started prepping some notes in early June. I am not a procrastinator and like to get things done as early as possible. The problem was I got so preoccupied with other things that I didn't look at them again until I was on the plane flying to D.C., which was the same day I had to speak. Not my smartest move.

In my defense, I had been at a horse show in Saugerties, New York the whole previous week, so I was pretty exhausted. A friend of mine was dying to see D.C., so we planned a whole speech for us to use to ask our parents if she could come. We told them that she was going to be my personal assistant. They both said yes, which was surprising, so she came with my mom and me on the trip.

I got home from Saugerties that Sunday night at 8pm, and my friend got dropped off at my house at 8:30pm because our flight was at 7am the next morning. The two of us were not happy campers waking up at 4am, but once we were up we were really excited. A driver picked us up at our house and we were off to the airport by 4:30 Monday morning.

After we had boarded the plane, there was a lot of traffic on the runway, so it took us an extra hour to takeoff. That is longer than the actual flight was! Nevertheless, we made it there by 10am, checked into the hotel, and grabbed some lunch. I had to be down in the lobby of the hotel at 2:30pm to speak at 3.

My mom is pretty adventurous and laid back, so we decided to take a walk around the city at 11am. It was 90 degrees out and I had already straightened my hair so I *really* didn't want to shower before speaking, because then I would have to blow out and straighten my hair all over again, which becomes an hour and a half ordeal. While walking around and exploring the city, my mom caught a glimpse of those Citi bikes that you can take out for an hour or however long you want. My mom being my mom, decided that it was a great idea. I was not in favor of this idea because it was already so hot and I wanted to go back to the hotel before I got super sweaty, besides the fact that my hair was getting frizzier by the minute. My mom ended up convincing me to take the bikes out for a little while, saying that afterwards we would go back to the hotel for me to put my makeup on and get ready to speak with plenty of time to spare. Talk about peer pressure.

We were having a blast riding those bikes around, but it was really freaking hot outside. I was wearing a white lace shirt and jeans (obviously not biking clothes as this was not part of the plan), and I remember feeling the sweat drip down my back (very sorry for that disgusting graphic imagery). So clearly now a shower was necessary before I went to speak to one hundred people. Then, of course of all times, my blood sugar went low. My vision was getting really blurry and I could barely walk in a straight line. And I still had this stupid bike. We went over to a little cart on the side of the road to get me a Coke. I chugged half of the bottle and then made it clear that it was time to find somewhere to put the bikes back because it was 2pm and I was supposed to be in the lobby in 30 minutes. Did I mention I still had to shower and redo my hair?!

I finally convinced my mom that it was really time to get back to the hotel. My mom agreed, so we brought our bikes back to where we got them. But when we got there, there were only two spots to return the bikes and we had three of them. We couldn't just leave the one bike there without locking it back in because it would've kept charging my mom's credit card until someone returned it. At this point it was 2:10pm, and I was practically having heart palpitations because I was so stressed (in case you didn't figure it out yet, I am a complete planner and like to get places at least ten minutes before I have to). My mom told me to walk back to the hotel and she would meet us there after she figured out what to do with this bike. My friend and I started walking, but realized we had no idea where to go. I am directionally challenged and she had never been to D.C. before, but thankfully navigation got us back to the hotel another ten minutes later.

When we got back to the hotel it was 2:20pm. I had to be in the lobby in ten minutes. These were obviously far from ideal circumstances. I took the fastest shower of my life and threw some makeup on, but I clearly didn't have time to blowout and straighten my hair. I had to improvise a little bit in that regard; I put it in a messy, disastrous looking bun and called it a day.

The way this event worked was that all of the delegates were coming down to this private room in the hotel where the speakers were set up. There were twelve speakers including myself, so each of us had our own table and we were instructed to bring props ahead of time. Since I was talking about riding, I brought my helmet, spurs, crop, some of my ribbons, and framed pictures. The delegates could choose which speeches they wanted to listen to. There were five rounds so I gave the same speech five times, fifteen minutes each.

I gathered all of my props, and headed down to the lobby. By the way, my mom was still not back by this point, so I was getting a little worried. I called her and she said she was walking back to the hotel. She had called the number on the machine and they said that she had to walk to a different location in order to stop her credit card from being charged, which is why it took her so long to get back. She took a quick shower and then came to help me set up my table.

After we got my table all set up, my friend and my mom went to Starbucks because I didn't want them to watch me present. I find that I can present better and be myself more when no one I know is watching me.

The head of Children's Congress came over the microphone once all of the delegates and their families arrived, and explained how the event was going to work. I was so nervous; I hadn't even looked at my notes before to think about what I was going to say. My first group that came over was mostly little kids with their parents, which made me feel better. I glanced at my notes every once in a while to make sure I was hitting all of the points I wanted to. I was so relieved when that first session was over! The next four were a breeze. After each one I got more and more confident and by the last one, I didn't even need my notes. My favorite part was how so many people came up to me and asked if I would take a picture with them. How cool is that? I felt like a celebrity!

My mom, my friend, and I went out for a celebratory dinner afterwards at an amazing Italian restaurant. Then, we went back to the hotel for an early night because our flight home was at 8am the next morning.

Just recently, I thought about all of my speaking opportunities so far and tried to decide which one I enjoyed the most. I came to the conclusion that it was Children's Congress in 2017. I think it was all of the kids that made me open up in a way that I never had before. Thinking back, I wonder if this was the event that made me lean more towards the pediatric side of endocrinology. I feel like it gave me the perfect platform to show the future victims of T1D that they are capable of doing anything they set their minds to no matter how difficult it may seem.

Like It's Not Hard Enough Already

One day a few years ago, underneath the adhesive of my pod was really itchy. I thought nothing of it, but it was just really annoying. It was the kind of terrible itching that keeps you up in the middle of the night. You know when you get five mosquito bites in a ten-centimeter radius and all you want to do is scratch? It was like that, except I couldn't scratch it because the part that was itchy was underneath the adhesive. The other strange part was that underneath my skin was rock-hard where the pod was. It seemed as though the insulin was being trapped underneath. I still don't know what it was for sure, but at the time, I was thinking perhaps I am allergic to the adhesive on the back of the pod. The lump that formed under my skin was painful as well. Just another enigma of Type 1.

The next day, I was due to change my pod. I disconnected it and ripped it off really fast (you have to do it super-fast like a band-aid otherwise it really hurts) and I kid you not, it was beet red with yellow puss coming out of it. If I stopped holding a paper towel over it, the yellow puss would drip everywhere. It was nasty (sorry for that disgustingly graphic description yet again. Now you're probably puking. Sorry about that). It was strange because it seemed like an open wound; it was raw, almost like I had ripped the skin right off. The worst part was that it hurt badly.

I found this bizarre; we thought it was just a one-time thing and that it wouldn't happen again. So I put a new pod on, but two days later I noticed that it was itching again underneath the adhesive. *Not again,* I thought to myself. I decided I was going to suck it up and wait until the next day when I was due to change it to see if it was the same issue. Sure enough, the exact same problem occurred. My dad called OnmiPod, the manufacturer, and asked them if they had changed their adhesive or anything in it. We took pictures of the reaction (or whatever you want to call it), and sent them to my endocrinologist. He said he thought I was allergic to something in the adhesive, but OmniPod claimed they hadn't changed anything. The whole thing was so bizarre.

It was leaving my body with so many bad scars on my arms and legs, so I could not go on using the pod if this was going to be the result. As much as I hated wearing the pump with tubing that I'd used before (the Animas), it seemed I didn't have much of a choice. My dad called to order a new updated Animas pump because the one I had was really old. They said that my insurance didn't cover a new pump for another two years, which was a major problem because pumps are REALLY expensive.

When we spoke to my endocrinologist about ways to stop this from happening, he recommended this serum that came as a wipe that you put on your skin before sticking the pod on; it formed a plastic-like barrier. That worked for about two weeks and then I became resistant to it. Once that stopped working, we tried a new method: we took a sticky piece of plastic and put that on prior to the pod so that when I stuck the pod on, it wasn't directly touching my skin at all. That worked for six months. Then, I started getting the rash again. It wasn't as bad as the initial reaction I had, but it still wasn't pleasant. Lately, I have been using the serum wipe prior to putting the plastic on before my pod. I guess we'll see how that works out.

Needless to say, this situation has been another big pain in the ass that has left scars everywhere. The scars that my pod and CGM have created all over my body are ugly, and I used to be very self-conscious of them. Some days I still am. But they are not something I can change, so I need to learn to cope with them. The days where I feel the most vulnerable are the ones where I'm wearing a bathing suit. Most other girls my age have beautiful skin with not a single blemish, but I have scars everywhere I look. But they serve a purpose. Those scars are my battle wounds, and they serve as a road map reminding me of everything I've been through that's gotten me to where I am today. Although they may not look pretty on the outside, they are a reminder that I have the strength to fight the fight every freaking day.

Max: Take 2

My dad came home from work one day with a message from the head of Stem for Life asking if my family would return to Italy in 2018 to speak at the conference again. He asked me my opinions and I said I had to think about it because it was my junior year of high school, so it would be difficult to miss a whole week of school. I don't like missing school because then you have to play catch-up when you get back, which totally stresses me out. Even when I'm sick or not feeling well, I try my hardest to go to school because I hate knowing that I will have work to make up when I get back.

A few weeks later, my dad said he needed my final decision. I told him that, unfortunately, I thought it would just be too hard to miss five days of school, and I therefore needed to pass up this opportunity. However, my dad was still planning on attending the conference because he was speaking on a few different panels again. He gave me a bit of a hard time about it, but he eventually respected my decision.

Two months later, I came home one afternoon to a very surprising conversation over dinner. My dad said that because I said no to come back to the Vatican, they wanted to do an interview closer to us (location-wise) for them to use at the conference.

However, this conversation was on a Tuesday, and that was when I found out that Max Gomez (who we'd previously met in Italy back in 2016) was going to be at my house with his camera man at 1pm that Friday. Now I'm someone who needs to mentally prepare for things. And you might be thinking, "Mentally prepare? You have three days to do that!" But I need a solid two weeks for something like this (yes, I know I'm a psycho). So at that point I was practically having a heart attack about my hair being a mess on camera, the fact that I had no idea what kinds of questions I was going to be asked, and that this whole thing was going to happen in just three days. I called the hair salon first thing the next morning and booked an appointment to get my hair blown out for Friday morning. I couldn't look like a mess if this was going to be filmed!

As the week went by in what felt like a flash, I was getting more and more nervous by the day. Caroline was also going to be speaking with me, so the plan was for me to pick her up from school at 12:00pm, come home so we could change and get cleaned up, and then we had to disappear for an hour because Max wanted to interview my parents alone first. My dad had told Max that we would be home at 2pm so we had to leave at 12:40pm to ensure that no one would see us ahead of time, since Max and his crew were told to come at 1pm. The plan was for Caroline and me to drive around aimlessly until 2pm, when we would then arrive home "straight from school."

Before I tell you what happened next, I need to explain something about my house. We have this alert system that we call "the beep," which basically beeps really loudly all around the house when a car pulls up our driveway, so we always know when someone arrives at our house. So it was 12:30pm, and we were getting all cleaned up and ready to go drive around when all of the sudden, the beep went off. Caroline and I looked at each other and flew out the door because we knew we were in trouble. The car I drive is always parked outside of the garage, which was the main problem. We had to pass whichever car just drove up the driveway in order to even get to the car. Caroline and I snuck out the back door and ran behind the shed. We thought that would be an easier route to the car without being seen. So here I am in jeans and a nice shirt with dress boots on in the snow, behind the shed. I counted to three and told Caroline that we were both going to sprint to the car. "1…2…3!" The two of us ran as fast as we could. However, there was a little hiccup in our plan, which happens to be hilarious for everyone except me. As I was running up the hill to get to the car, I started slipping in the snow because it was at that stage where it was slushy and starting to melt. It was especially slippery considering I was in dress boots. Right as I felt myself slipping, I grabbed the ground with my hands because the last thing I needed at this point was to fall in the slush and get wet. My feet started slipping out from under me; I looked like a hamster running on one of those little wheels. I just couldn't recover! Long story short, I fell in the slush. Exactly what I needed. I got up and hopped in the car with my pants soaking wet. Mental note…never wear cute boots in the snow. Snow boots only.

Anyway, we managed to escape because it was only the camera guy. I timed it so we were driving out of the driveway when he was bringing all of his equipment inside the house. After that, we drove around with no destination for an hour and a half. Max was mid-interview with my parents when we arrived back at our house at 2pm. We came in quietly, but I got into a laughing fit and couldn't stop while my mom was talking, so Caroline and I got kicked out of the kitchen. We were banished from the first floor and had to go upstairs until it was our turn.

Once it was finally time for us to be interviewed, we went downstairs and had our microphones put on. We were interviewed and filmed for about an hour and a half. Once I got comfortable, it was actually a lot of fun. Max hung out for a bit afterwards and he really is such an amazing and kind person.

Although it was short notice, it was great being able to shoot some video footage for the Stem for Life Conference. Their mission is so important, and I am thrilled to do whatever it takes to improve the quality of life for everyone living with Type 1. The more awareness we raise, the more people we have on our side to help us fight, and in this case, the more the merrier.

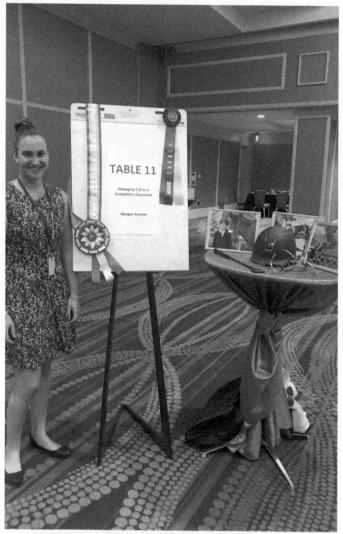

Children's Congress 2017 where I spoke at the first event of the weekend. This was my table that I prepared.

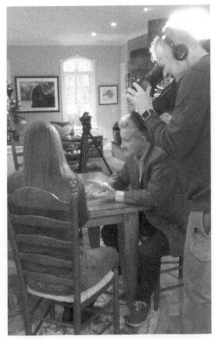

Our interview with Max in the works.
Don't mind our Christmas decorations!

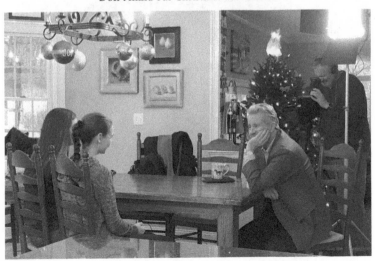

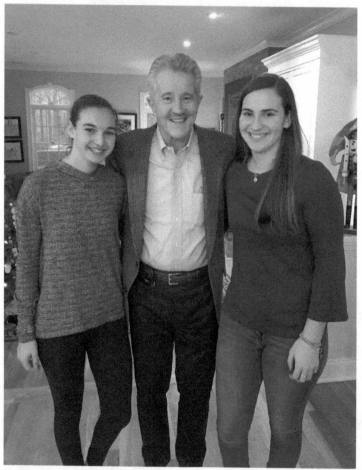

Caroline, Max and me after filming our interview in December of 2017.

Part VI

"When you can't change the direction of the wind,

adjust your sails."

H. JACKSON BROWN

Haters Gonna Hate

Throughout my life, I have encountered many people who don't support me. During my freshman year of high school, I was verbally bullied. I was told that Type 1 was a joke and wasn't a big deal by people who have zero connection to and knowledge of T1D whatsoever. These same people said they had no idea why I was even invited to speak in Italy because there was no reason to and that it was pointless. This nonsense went on for weeks, and it got to the point where I would end up in my guidance counselor's office and go home in tears almost every day.

There have also been people who have told me that writing this book was stupid and a waste of time. They said that no one cared about my life. That's fine, maybe it's true. But if by sharing my story I can cause just one person on this Earth to feel empowered or continue fighting this fight, then it was worth it.

At the end of the day, these individuals served as a lesson for me. They taught me that there are always going to be people in your life who don't support you and constantly want to bring you down. And there are various reasons for this. Maybe they are arrogant, maybe they are jealous, or maybe they are just that type of person. But no matter what the real reason is, we can't get upset over it. We should use these types of people as motivators. In most cases it's just not worth arguing with them. Instead, the best revenge is to do exactly what they said you couldn't and more. If someone tells you you can't run one mile, run two. As sad as it sounds, your success will piss them off more than anything else in the world.

The Teenage Years

Being a teenager is tough enough, but throw Type 1 into the mix and things can get ugly if you don't take care of yourself. I remember when I was ten or eleven, my dad sat me down and talked to me about the complications of T1D. It was during this same conversation that he brought something very important to my attention. He said that often times when people with Type 1 get to be teenagers and even into their twenties, they stop taking care of themselves. This shocked me; there was never a moment that I thought about stopping to take care of myself altogether. To me, that meant ending my life which was simply not an option. When I asked him why on Earth anyone would ever do this, he said it's because they didn't want other people to know they had T1D. He told me that he heard stories of people going on dates and just not bolusing for food at all because he/she was scared to expose his/her illness to the other person. He also said that a lot of people will intentionally not give themselves insulin with the hope that their blood sugar will stay extremely high, because having such severe hyperglycemia causes weight loss. Hearing both of these things made me sad and discouraged.

This conversation really made me think about a lot of different things, but it mostly made me wonder how I could help stop this problem. The complications of Type 1 are absolutely horrific, and there is no way that I would ever jeopardize my health to impress someone or even to lose weight. I understand that the teenage years are tough, and often times we do anything we can to fit in. But sometimes fitting in isn't the best option. Instead of trying to hide Type 1, I've decided to show the world that I have it. I've embraced it. I challenge you to do the same. If someone doesn't want to date you, or be friends with you, or whatever the circumstance may be only because you have Type 1, then that person doesn't deserve to know you and all that you offer.

Actually, I Can.

I know I already told you this story, but when I was in the hospital getting rabies shots, because there had been a bat in our house, the nurse came in to give us, or should I say Caroline and Luke, ice pops. She said to them, "Here you go!" Then when she got to me she said, "Oh sorry, you can't have one. They aren't sugar free."

Actually, I can.

To the ones who think that I can't play sports as well as you can because I have Type 1.
Well guess what?

Actually, I can.

To those who think I am not as smart as others because my disease affects me mentally. To those same people that think I'm not capable of getting As.

Actually, I can.

To all of the people who think I can't eat candy, cupcakes, cake, brownies, and any other sweet you can have, because I have T1D.

Actually, I can.

To anyone who thinks that because I am only one person, I don't have the ability to make a change for me and for all of those suffering from Type 1.

Actually, I can.

Looking Ahead

As I wrote this book, it really forced me to think about my goals, dreams, and what I want to do in the future. I know I've mentioned it before, but I have decided that I want to be a pediatric endocrinologist who specializes in Type 1 diabetes. While practicing as a doctor, I also would love to go around the world advocating on behalf of all people with Type 1 because I feel that T1D is viewed by the general public as just a simple disease that stinks, but if you take a pill once a day, you'll be fine. I want to show people that this isn't nearly as simple as taking a pill. I wish it were. I would like to be able to make an impact and help everyone suffering from T1D.

I also want to be able to show my fellow fighters that this disease won't limit you as long as you don't let it. And for anyone who doesn't have T1D, I want to show them that guess what? I can do anything you can do. It won't stop me.

One of my dreams, I have already accomplished. Ever since I started writing this book years ago, I really wanted to get it out to the public. I took a lot of breaks, and I cannot tell you how many times I almost deleted it from my computer altogether. I almost gave up. But then one day, I decided that this is a disease that people need to understand. The misconceptions need to end.

I always thought of myself as just some normal teenage girl who did normal teenage things: went to school, had a hobby that I loved (riding), hung out with friends, ate, and slept. I never thought I would have the ability to make a change in the Type 1 diabetes world. But I am absolutely humbled and thrilled that I have been able to advocate to all of the people that I have. Who knew by age eighteen I would have met...

Pope Francis

Martha Stewart

Max Gomez

Dean Kamen

Jared Allen

Sugar Ray Leonard

Nick Jonas

Robin Roberts

Katie Couric

Gary Hall Jr.

Joe Biden

Barack Obama

Never in a million years would I have pictured myself advocating to all of the influential people that I have. From being on Martha Stewart's show to speaking in Vatican City and receiving the Pontifical Hero Award from Pope Francis, I am truly flattered to have had such incredible opportunities, and to have met all of the amazing people that I have. I look forward to continuing to fight and creating a new way of thinking about "diabetes" on behalf of everyone fighting Type 1.

The Comeback

Over the years, I have learned so much about myself, strength, bravery, and life in general. I say this being completely honest: I thank God for giving me T1D for two reasons. One: so someone else in the world doesn't have to endure it, and two: because it has made me a much stronger person than I ever could have been without it. I don't let it limit me because if it does, what's life worth? It would win, and with this miserable disease, you want to come out on top.

I go to bed every night wondering if I'll wake up in the morning due to a fatal high or low blood sugar. As it's an extremely dangerous disease, Type 1 has taught me nothing less than to live every day to the fullest. It has made me appreciate every hour, every minute, and every second I stand on this Earth. But the truth is everyone should live this way, because you don't know if you'll receive life-changing news tomorrow, and you don't know if today is your last day. Everyone has obstacles in their lives; it's just the way life is. But you don't have to sit there and let them beat you down.

Defeat them. Strength is a choice, and if you tell yourself you can get through whatever you're battling, then you can.

I could not be more thankful that Type 1 has put things into perspective for me. If nothing else, it has made me more thankful and stronger than ever.

I also never understood why people tried to hide it. This is part of who I am, and why would I try to hide it if I have no choice? It will be with me for the rest of my life, so I've decided to embrace it. Be proud of yourself for conquering this and say, "Yes I am a Type 1 diabetic, and you shouldn't mess with me because look at this hell that I go through every day that I call my life. And look how much tougher it's made me."

The, "Oh my life sucks because I have this disease" attitude is not the one to live by. It is so much more empowering to think about it this way: "Yes this disease sucks, it is such a pain in the ass, and has had such an impact on my everyday life, but look at the kind of person it's made me." Make it into a positive. Not everything in your life has to be negative all of the time. This was something I had to learn because I was, like most, only seeing the negative. Just remember: there's always a positive. No matter how deep it's buried, I promise you it's there. There is a reason that you're in the situation you are right now. Whether it's to better yourself or educate others, there is reasoning behind it. You may not understand why your life is hell now, but you will later. You have to trust me on that.

I really appreciate you allowing me to share my journey with you, but I have one last piece of advice. Something I learned along the way, and it took me way too long to figure out. So I will share it with you so you don't have to spend your life searching for answers like I did. No matter what you are going through, whether it be hell or high water, just remember this: if I can get through it, so can you. You're a winner. Beat whatever you're battling. Show your "something" that you will come out on top no matter what it takes, and don't let it get the best of you. If you rally through the hard times, things will get better. I've shared my story, now it's your turn to share yours. Most importantly, in times of doubt, turn your struggle into strength and always remember, "Actually, you can."

Thanks for reading!

- Morgan

Acknowledgements

I first want to thank my parents, who have been there for me every step of the way, and have supported me since day one. Whether it is waking up at all hours of the night to check my blood sugar, helping me achieve my goal of publishing a book, or anything in between, they have been through it all. I could not be more blessed to have these two amazing people in my life. Mom and dad, you are not only my favorite people, but my best friends. I will always wonder how I got so lucky. I love you both so much, and nothing will ever suffice in thanking you for all you have done for me.

I also want to thank my sister, Caroline and my brother, Luke. Thanks for being my rocks and always keeping me in check. You guys are the absolute best. I love you and am so proud of you both.

To my grandma, Mimi, the most loving and generous person I know. Thank you for setting the best example for me. I could not have asked for a better role model to have growing up. You will be my hero forever.

To my best friend, Rachel. Thank you for everything you do to make me laugh and keep me going. It's people like you who help me continue to fight this battle.

Finally, I want to say a huge thank-you to my high school English teacher, Karen Zlotnick. Karen is someone who greatly assisted me throughout this process. When I was at a point where I was feeling discouraged and didn't know where, if anywhere, this book was going to go, she read it and encouraged me to stick with it. Karen made me feel like my message was worth sharing with others. She is one of my biggest supporters, and is someone who has impacted my life in a profound way. Karen, thank you so much for all of your motivation and support. You are one of the main reasons why I was able to get to where I am today, and I am forever grateful for everything you have done for me.